Thoracic Surgical Education: Current and Future Strategies

Editor

EDWARD D. VERRIER

THORACIC SURGERY CLINICS

www.thoracic.theclinics.com

Consulting Editor
M. BLAIR MARSHALL

August 2019 • Volume 29 • Number 3

ELSEVIER

1600 John F. Kennedy Boulevard • Suite 1800 • Philadelphia, Pennsylvania, 19103-2899

http://www.thoracic.theclinics.com

THORACIC SURGERY CLINICS Volume 29, Number 3
August 2019 ISSN 1547-4127, ISBN-13: 978-0-323-68251-0

Editor: John Vassallo (j.vassallo@elsevier.com)
Developmental Editor: Laura Fisher

Thoracic Surgery Clinics (ISSN 1547-4127) is published quarterly by Elsevier Inc., 360 Park Avenue South, New York, NY 10010-1710. Months of publication are February, May, August, and November. Business and editorial offices: 1600 John F. Kennedy Boulevard, Suite 1800, Philadelphia, PA 19103-2899. Periodicals postage paid at New York, NY, and additional mailing offices. Subscription prices are $382.00 per year (US individuals), $585.00 per year (US institutions), $100.00 per year (US students), $460.00 per year (Canadian individuals), $757.00 per year (Canadian institutions), $225.00 per year (Canadian and international students), $475.00 per year (international individuals), and $757.00 per year (international institutions). Foreign air speed delivery is included in all Clinics' subscription prices. All prices are subject to change without notice. **POSTMASTER:** Send address changes to Thoracic Surgery Clinics, Elsevier Health Sciences Division, Subscription Customer Service, 3251 Riverport Lane, Maryland Heights, MO 63043. **Customer Service (orders, claims, online, change of address): Telephone: 1-800-654-2452 (U.S. and Canada); 314-447-8871 (outside U.S. and Canada). Fax: 314-447-8029. E-mail: journalscustomerservice-usa@elsevier.com (for print support); journalsonlinesupport-usa@elsevier.com (for online support).**

Reprints. For copies of 100 or more, of articles in this publication, please contact Commercial Rights Department, Elsevier Inc., 360 Park Avenue South, New York, NY 10010-1710. Tel: 212-633-3874; Fax: 212-633-3820; E-mail: reprints@elsevier.com.

Thoracic Surgery Clinics is covered in *MEDLINE/PubMed (Index Medicus), EMBASE/Excerpta Medica, Science Citation Index Expanded (SciSearch®), Journal Citation Reports/Science Edition,* and *Current Contents®/Clinical Medicine.*

Contributors

CONSULTING EDITOR

M. BLAIR MARSHALL, MD, FACS
Chief, Division of Thoracic Surgery, Associate
Professor, Department of Surgery,
Georgetown University Medical Center,
Georgetown University School of Medicine,
Washington, DC, USA

EDITOR

EDWARD D. VERRIER, MD
K Alvin Merendino Professor of Cardiovascular
Surgery, Division of Cardiothoracic Surgery,
Department of Surgery, University
of Washington, Seattle, Washington,
USA

AUTHORS

LAUREN ALOIA, BA
Former Employee of The Society of Thoracic
Surgeons and The Joint Council of Thoracic
Surgery Education, Jupiter, Florida, USA

LEAH M. BACKHUS, MD, MPH
Stanford University, Stanford, California, USA

KATHLEEN BERFIELD, MD
Assistant Professor, Department of Surgery,
Division of CT Surgery, University of
Washington, UWMC, Seattle, Washington,
USA

ERROL L. BUSH, MD
Johns Hopkins School of Medicine, Johns
Hopkins University, Baltimore, Maryland,
USA

**CHRISTOPHER CAO, MBBS, BSc, PhD,
FRACS**
Department of Cardiothoracic Surgery, NYU
Langone Health, New York, New York, USA;
Department of Cardiothoracic Surgery, Royal
Prince Alfred Hospital, Sydney, New South
Wales, Australia

**ROBERT J. CERFOLIO, MD, MBA, FACS,
FCCP**
Senior Vice President and Vice Dean,
Chief Operating Officer, Professor of
Cardiothoracic Surgery, Chief of Clinical
Thoracic Surgery, Director of Lung Cancer
Center, Department of Cardiothoracic Surgery,
NYU Langone Health, New York, New York,
USA

DAVID T. COOKE, MD
UC Davis Medical Center, University of
California, Sacramento, Sacramento,
California, USA

JOSEPH A. DEARANI, MD
Professor of Surgery, Department
of Cardiovascular Surgery, Mayo
Clinic, Rochester, Minnesota,
USA

ZACHARY ENUMAH, MD
Johns Hopkins School of Medicine, Johns
Hopkins University, Baltimore, Maryland,
USA

JAMES I. FANN, MD
Professor, Department of Cardiothoracic
Surgery, Stanford University, Stanford,
California, USA

JOSHUA L. HERMSEN, MD
Assistant Professor of Surgery, Division of
Cardiothoracic Surgery, University of
Wisconsin-Madison and American
Family Children's Hospital, Madison,
Wisconsin, USA

ROBERT HIGGINS, MD, MSHA
Johns Hopkins School of Medicine,
Johns Hopkins University, Baltimore,
Maryland, USA

AMY L. HOLMSTROM, MD
Department of Surgery, Northwestern
University Feinberg School of Medicine,
Chicago, Illinois, USA

JULES LIN, MD
Mark B. Orringer Professor, Associate
Professor, Section of Thoracic Surgery,
University of Michigan Medical Center, Ann
Arbor, Michigan, USA

NATALIE S. LUI, MD, MAS
Stanford University, Stanford, California, USA

DOUGLAS J. MATHISEN, MD
Chief, Thoracic Surgery, Massachusetts
General Hospital, Boston, Massachusetts,
USA

SHARI L. MEYERSON, MD, MEd
Department of Surgery, University of Kentucky,
Lexington, Kentucky, USA

NAHUSH A. MOKADAM, MD, FACS, FACC
Professor and Director, Kakos and Williams
Endowed Professor in Cardiac Surgery,
Division of Cardiac Surgery, Department
of Surgery, The Ohio State University Wexner
Medical Center, Columbus, Ohio, USA

CHRISTOPHER R. MORSE, MD
Thoracic Surgery, Massachusetts General
Hospital, Boston, Massachusetts, USA

RISHINDRA M. REDDY, MD
Jose Alvarez Professor, Associate Professor,
Section of Thoracic Surgery, Surgery Clerkship
Director, University of Michigan Medical
Center, Ann Arbor, Michigan, USA

PHILLIP G. ROWSE, MD
Assistant Professor of Surgery, Department of
Cardiovascular Surgery, Mayo Clinic,
Rochester, Minnesota, USA

GREGORY D. RUSHING, MD
Assistant Professor, Division of Cardiac
Surgery, Department of Surgery, The Ohio
State University Wexner Medical Center,
Columbus, Ohio, USA

AHMAD Y. SHEIKH, MD
Staff Physician, Division of Cardiothoracic
Surgery, Kaiser Permanente, Assistant Clinical
Professor, Division of Cardiothoracic Surgery,
University of California, San Francisco, San
Francisco, California, USA

ARA A. VAPORCIYAN, MD, FACS, MHPE
Professor and Chair, Department of Thoracic
and Cardiovascular Surgery, The University of
Texas MD Anderson Cancer Center, Houston,
Texas, USA

EDWARD D. VERRIER, MD
K Alvin Merendino Professor of Cardiovascular
Surgery, Division of Cardiothoracic Surgery,
Department of Surgery, University of
Washington, Seattle, Washington, USA

STEPHEN C. YANG, MD
The Arthur B. and Patricia B. Modell Endowed
Chair in Thoracic Surgery, Professor of Surgery
and Oncology, Division of Thoracic Surgery,
The Johns Hopkins Medical Institutions,
Baltimore, Maryland, USA

Contents

Surgical education in 2019 faces may challenges to maintain the high standards of excellence achieved in prior generations of learners and trainers in cardiothoracic surgery. This compendium hopes to review the current and future strategies in surgical education. The topics include the adult learner, assessing competence, providing formative feedback, developing strategies to minimize implicit bias, optimizing education in the operating room, effective classroom teaching, the future of e-learning, the alternative curriculum, teaching mentorship and coaching, deliberate practice and simulation, faculty development, the potential roles of virtual and augmented reality, and the impact artificial intelligence might have on surgical education in the future.

Both the breadth of knowledge and range of technical skills that residents are now expected to master prior to graduation have grown exponentially. A unique challenge that sets surgical education apart from medical education is that surgery as a specialty requires not only the mastery of complex physiology, anatomy, and disease processes but also the ability to interpret and apply that knowledge In the operating room. To be effective educators, it is imperative to understand the theoretic foundation of how adults learn.

Training in thoracic surgery has evolved immensely over the past decade due to the advent of integrated programs, technological innovations, and regulations on resident duty hours, decreasing the time trainees have to learn. These changes have made assessment of thoracic surgical trainees even more important. Shifts in medical education have increasingly emphasized competency, which has led to novel competency-based assessment tools for clinical and operative assessment. These novel tools take advantage of simulation and modern technology to provide more frequent and comprehensive assessment of the surgical trainee to ensure competence.

Unfortunately, evidence-based models of formative feedback are rare in graduate medical education. Adapting models developed in K-12 learning is a surrogate but with some exceptions. One of these models is presented in the context of thoracic surgical education. Its utility is demonstrated when delivering formative feedback. The recognized few but key differences between K-12 education and graduate medical education regarding how feedback works are highlighted. These can limit feedback's effectiveness and so suggestions from the literature to avoid their impact are offered. The work is summarized with a set of guidelines to help in the delivery of formative feedback.

Unconscious (or implicit) biases are learned stereotypes that are automatic, unintentional, deeply engrained, universal, and able to influence behavior. Several studies have documented the effects of provider biases on patient care and outcomes. This article provides a framework for exploring the implications for unconscious bias in surgical education and highlights best practices toward minimizing its impact. Presented is the background related to some of the more common unconscious biases and effects on medical students, resident trainees, and academic faculty. Finally, targeted strategies are highlighted for individuals and institutions for identification of biases and the means to address them.

Resident education in the operating room and surgical resident autonomy represent two enormous challenges within cardiothoracic (CT) training programs. The goal of surgical educators and CT trainees is to ensure the graduating resident's ability to safely operate independently at the completion of training. The field has come a long way from the notion of see one, do one, teach one, which was once the norm. Cardiothoracic surgery continues to become more specialized and the patients more complex with greater scrutiny of outcomes. There are many challenges that are faced in contemporary CT training to make intraoperative teaching harder than ever.

Classic classroom education emphasizes the teacher imparting knowledge, experience, or wisdom (pedagogy). Adult educational theory indicates learning is optimized in an experiential setting, where the learner prepares, the session is case based, and the responsibility of the educator is to teach what the learner does not know. This is referred to as "flipping the classroom." Flipping the classroom is not simple, as the historical educational culture often changes; and, at least early in the transition process, different expectations, preparation, or training are essential for both the learner and educator for this approach to be effective.

Education in all fields is vastly different today than it was 20 years ago. Constraints on time, access to clinical material and the speed of change mandate new more efficient approaches to education. Today, the Internet is a powerful tool that students and educators use to supplement or replace traditional learning. This technique, referred to as E-learning, can deliver a broad array of solutions that enhance knowledge and performance. We review some of the current applications of E-learning in cardiothoracic surgery and suggest some future applications that may further enhance the efficiency of cardiothoracic surgical education.

Stephen C. Yang

Surgical training has focused on the development of technical competency. Inter-personal and cognitive skills are essential to working as an interdisciplinary team, which translates into safety for the patient and well-being for the surgeon and colleagues. This article offers an "alternative" surgical curriculum topic list to augment the technical skill sets traditionally taught to trainees.

Phillip G. Rowse and Joseph A. Dearani

In the current era of duty hour limitations and societal focus on cardiothoracic sur-gical outcomes, simulation and deliberate practice have emerged as valuable sup-plemental training options. Evidence supporting acquisition of technical skill, clinical transferability, and patient safety within the realm of simulation is mounting. This article provides a focused synthesis of evidence regarding the usefulness of simulation-based training and deliberate practice as a whole and within the subspe-cialty of cardiothoracic surgery.

Jules Lin and Rishindra M. Reddy

Teaching and mentorship have a long history in surgical education, but with a growing focus on safety, quality improvement, and continuous professional development, it is clear that the current training system is inadequate. Challenges from changes in res-idency training, financial constraints, rapidly increasing knowledge, and limited faculty time due to increasing clinical, academic, and research demands require that new ap-proaches are developed, including simulation and online resources. Although coach-ing is used effectively in other disciplines, surgical coaching remains relatively uncommon. Coaching encourages self-reflection using facilitated feedback individu-alized to each surgeon's needs and goals and can benefit surgeons at all levels.

Gregory D. Rushing and Nahush A. Mokadam

Faculty development is important at any level of academic rank but is especially important in early stages. The clinical educator is a rewarding pathway that is emerging as a special track for promotion and advancement. Success is achievable through development of skills, measurement of progress, obtaining funding, and completion of projects through publication. Advanced degrees, mentorship, and persistence are keys to achievement.

Christopher Cao and Robert J. Cerfolio

Virtual reality and augmented reality technologies have evolved with a growing pres-ence in both clinical care and surgical training.

Artificial intelligence (AI) is being rapidly integrated into various medical applications. Although early application of AI has been achieved in image-based, as well as statistical computational models, translation into procedure-based specialties such as surgery may take longer to achieve. A potential application of AI in surgical education is as a teaching coach or mentor that interacts with the used via virtual and/or augmented reality. The question arises as to whether machines will achieve the wisdom and intelligence of human educators.

THORACIC SURGERY CLINICS

SERIES OF RELATED INTEREST

Surgical Clinics
http://www.surgical.theclinics.com
Surgical Oncology Clinics
http://www.surgonc.theclinics.com
Advances in Surgery
http://www.advancessurgery.com

THE CLINICS ARE AVAILABLE ONLINE!
Access your subscription at:
www.theclinics.com

Preface
Fulfilling a Need

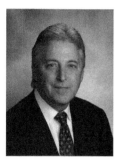

Edward D. Verrier, MD
Editor

We believe that resident surgical education in 2019 is being challenged both in and outside the operating room. Optimal outcomes are essential. Safety must be emphasized. Efficiency is paramount. Residents have duty-hour restrictions, and there is simply a malalignment of incentives distracting faculty. Expertise is not transferable across domains, and because one is an excellent academic or clinical surgeon does not mean they are excellent surgical educators without training. The responsibility to educate and train the next generation of surgeons is an essential responsibility to society. Surgical volume and complexity are increasing at a time when historically, the simpler cases, which for many years formed the basis of surgical training, are no longer done by surgeons. How do we not only maintain the historical excellence in surgical training we have come to know but actually improve? How do we implement educational advances in adult learning, understand bias, use deliberate practice, advance simulation, and then engage in the new educational opportunities provided by virtual reality and artificial intelligence? Maybe most importantly we hope to stimulate a new generation of educators who can contribute academically for their own career development and the improvement of surgical training in general. This issue hopes to fulfill a need concerning surgical education by changing the conversation and providing insight into current surgical training algorithms and evolving potentials for the future. We hope there is value in this issue beyond cardiothoracic surgery.

Edward D. Verrier, MD
Division of Cardiothoracic Surgery
Department of Surgery
University of Washington
1959 NE Pacific Street
Box 356310
Seattle, WA 98919, USA

E-mail address:
edver@uw.edu

Thorac Surg Clin 29 (2019) xi
https://doi.org/10.1016/j.thorsurg.2019.05.001
1547-4127/19/© 2019 Published by Elsevier Inc.

thoracic.theclinics.com

The Surgeon as Educator

Edward D. Verrier, MD

KEYWORDS

• Surgery • Resident • Education

KEY POINTS

- This article hopes to be a sentinel reference for cardiothoracic surgery educators, faculty, and residents.
- This compendium also hopes to stimulate academic interest for education research in cardiothoracic surgery.
- Surgical education.
- Improving Surgical faculty as educators.
- The future of surgical education in cardiothoracic surgery.

The effective teacher, more than anyone else, has the opportunity to affect eternity.
—Owen Wangensteen

Thoracic Surgery Clinics, under the editorial leadership of M. Blair Marshall, MD, has elected to put together a series of articles on the current state of cardiothoracic surgical education. This issue has been titled "Thoracic Surgery Education: Current and Future Strategies." Dr Marshall turned to the past leadership of the Joint Council on Thoracic Surgical Education, who for 10 years worked to improve the state of cardiothoracic surgical resident education to help with this effort.[1] In approaching the task of critically looking at resident education starting in 2008, the JCTSE team attempted to pool surgical educational expertise inside and outside cardiothoracic surgery, define necessary learning objectives, develop curriculum, institute content and learning management systems that could apply e-learning principles to resident education, transform classic written content from text books into interactive digital media, and emphasize overall faculty development as educators. The overarching goal was to raise awareness that surgical education was not simply an art form and avocation but rather a science and vocation that required study and commitment to do

well. Expertise is not transferable across domain and that simply because you are a good surgeon does not equate that you are also a good educator; to be a master educator one must actually study and work at it every day[2,3] (**Fig. 1**). In this issue on the current state of surgical education in cardiothoracic surgery, the authors have invited 14 leaders to put together authorship teams to discuss potentially important areas of surgical education pertinent to the current educational challenges In surgery.

Each of the investigators has been challenged not only to understand historical perspectives and review the current state of the art but also to look forward to suggest constructive, creative, and sustainable ways to improve educational environments in cardiothoracic surgery for the future, which is not a simple task.

HISTORICAL PERSPECTIVES

Our modern educational foundations in medicine and surgery date back to the turn of the twentieth century in the Johns Hopkins University tradition. Abraham Flexner was commissioned by the Carnegie Commission to look at medical education in the United States and Canada. His "Flexner" report was published in 1910 and concluded that

Disclosure: The author has nothing to disclose.
Division of Cardiothoracic Surgery, Department of Surgery, University of Washington, 8479 Woodland Cove Drive, Kirkland, WA 98034, USA
E-mail address: edver@uw.edu

Thorac Surg Clin 29 (2019) 227–232
https://doi.org/10.1016/j.thorsurg.2019.03.001
1547-4127/19/© 2019 Elsevier Inc. All rights reserved.

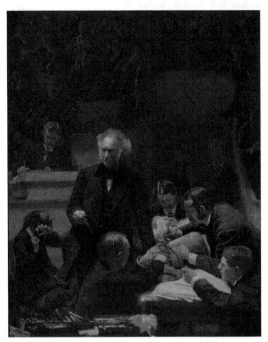

Fig. 1. The effective educator. Portrait of Dr Samuel D. Gross (The Gross Clinic) by Thomas Eakins. (Philadelphia Museum of Art, Gift of the Alumni Association to Jefferson Medical College in 1878 and purchased by the Pennsylvania Academy of the Fine Arts and the Philadelphia Museum of Art in 2007 with the generous support of more than 3,600 donors, 2007-1-1.)

prerequisite medical education must include high school and at least 2 years of university.[4] Medical school would then be 4 years with 2 basic preclinical years and 2 years of clinical clerkships. This would then be followed by variable postgraduate medical training in specific areas of medical or surgical expertise. This evolved then into the residency training algorithm, which first came under the American Board of Medical Specialties (1933), then ultimately came under the Accreditation Council of Graduate Medical Education (1981). Around the same time as Flexner was at Hopkins, William Halsted (1903) also at Hopkins outlined the principles of surgical education: first formalize the classic apprenticeship model, base surgery on scientific foundations, provide graded responsibility to trainees, define a reproducible structure, standardize training as much as possible, and create a competitive pyramidal schema.[5] William Osler next expanded the concepts by encouraging residents to work together but be supervised by competent, trained faculty with an emphasis on beside and operative teaching (1908). Later, Edward Churchill recommended a rectangular rather than pyramidal system and that model essentially persists till today (1933).[6]

Over a century later the foundations of medical and surgical education have minimally changed. In contrast, think about societal changes that have occurred over this past century. We have gone through 2 societal revolutions and 4 generations. We have progressed from the Model T automobile to the Tesla, from the airplane to rockets, from the printing press to the personal computer, and from the telephone to the Internet. Surgical practice has also evolved. There has been a logarithmic rather than linear growth in knowledge, we have moved from the era of reporting to the era of regulation. Innovation and creativity are being harnessed by patient safety and internal review boards. We are increasingly being measured by hospital financial bottom lines. Surgical efficiency is paramount. We have more potential or real conflicts with industry. Our outcome data are now transparent and reported. We have moved from small faculty with large volumes to large faculties with small volumes and increased subspecialization, and of course we have significant resident duty hour restrictions. Yet, our approach to surgical education has not substantially changed over this century.[2] When operative complexity was less, exposure was repetitive, immersion was expected, and the apprentice model was championed, the resulting resident product was usually ready for clinical practice and subsequently successful. When patient and surgical complexity went way up, new technology altered basic options, competition emerged from other medical specialties, time in the hospital for training went way down, and the emphasis had to shift from a simply time-based algorithm of training suited for all into one that placed the emphasis on "competency-based training" that would prepare a resident in the new practice environment of 2020.[7] The challenge then, of course, is that residents provide a substantial component of clinical service to academic medical centers, so the reality is that resident education remains time based and the ability to assess true cognitive or technical skill competency remains a challenge.[8]

CURRENT BROAD EDUCATIONAL CHALLENGES

It should be emphasized that education in general from kindergarten through medical school has been going through a complex analysis that sounds somewhat familiar to the one just described in surgery or medicine. All children do not learn in the same way or at the same rate or with the same emphasis (visual, auditory, tactile), so the concept of a graded set of classrooms that apply to a diverse population of learners is being challenged.[9] The teacher-centric approach to learning is also in some disfavor as if the learner is some sort of sponge (pedagogy) and we as educators simply play the role of dumping our wisdom or experience or knowledge on them and they will learn. This then becomes increasingly important in the adult learner who already has a learning foundation (family, societal, formalized educational, or professional) on which we must build to achieve this goal of competency and eventual surgical autonomy (andragogy).[10] First the adult learner makes a choice in what they want to learn and if they want to learn. Secondly, each adult learner has a style of learning and a unique pace. Finally, most adult learners need learning to be experiential and not passive in order to be effective. This reflects Kolb cycle, whereby one performs a task and then is given the opportunity to reflect on that task with accurate assessment and meaningful feedback, identifying areas where improvements can be made and then adjusting to the new cycle.[11] This has then led to the important evolving concepts of becoming learner-centric in education with its important consequences (what is called the constructivist theory of learning).[12] Basic principles include the following:

- Presence is not a substitute for active participation in the process of learning.
- The learner has to take significant responsibility in their own learning process (even more important than ever in the duty hour restricted model of resident education).
- Effective learning is not simply cramming short term or working memory with facts; it represents developing imagery in long-term memory that can be recalled effectively.[13]
- Active learning should stimulate higher-order thinking, problem solving, decision-making, and critical thinking, all crucial cognitive skills for the surgeon.
- The effective educator must hone critical assessment skills and learn how to provide meaningful, effective feedback.
- Teaching motor skills requires deliberate practice to achieve expertise.[14]
- Deliberate practice in skill acquisition involves the performer getting great at high-impact fundamental skills through repetition but also allows the learner to overlearn so the proficiency becomes second nature, cross-train to develop complimentary skills, and devise safe simulations to allow performance without fear.[2]
- The teacher-centric didactic teaching algorithm can be improved by learning how to use case-based learning approaches—what is now commonly referred to as "flipping the classroom."[15]

- Audiovisual learning is a science involving more than outdated, stale, bullet point–laden PowerPoint presentations.[16]
- Electronic learning management systems (with assessment and feedback) can be an effective adjunct to didactic or classroom learning in residency training.[1]
- Teaching, mentorship, and coaching are all necessary to achieve effective learning in the adult and they are not all the same.[2]

Many of these basic concepts are developed in significantly more detail in this issue.

THE QUEST FOR EXPERTISE—THE QUEST FOR AUTONOMY—THE QUEST TO SET THE FOUNDATIONS FOR LIFE-LONG LEARNING AND CONTINUAL IMPROVEMENT

The Dreyfus model of skill acquisition is a model of how learners acquire skills through instruction and practice. The model proposes that a student passes through 6 distinct phases: novice, advanced beginner, competence, proficiency, expertise, and mastery, and this is based on 4 binary qualities: recollection, recognition, decision, and awareness[17] (**Fig. 2**). In fact, the Dreyfus scale has commonly been applied to surgical education and is part of the foundation that led to this concept of "competency based medical education" adopted by the ACGME. Competency-based medical education (CBME) is an approach to preparing physicians for practice that is fundamentally oriented to graduate outcome abilities and organized around competencies derived from an analysis of societal and patient needs. It deemphasizes time-based training and promises greater accountability, flexibility, and learner-centeredness.[18] The ACGME has adopted 6 basic competencies: patient care, medical knowledge, professionalism, interpersonal and communication skills, practice-based learning and improvement, and system-based practice.[19] The application and implementation of CBME with achievement of competency defined "milestones" is the basis of evaluating all residency training programs in the United States and is rapidly being adopted around the world for training program accreditation. In the application of these concepts every day in surgical training, we then must look at our end points as educators and how we assess or measure such milestones and how we train faculty to achieve a similar degree of competency in their assessment and feedback skills. This thought then leads to the discussion of how we further define competency, proficiency, expertise, and mastery on that Dreyfus model of cognitive and skills acquisition in surgical

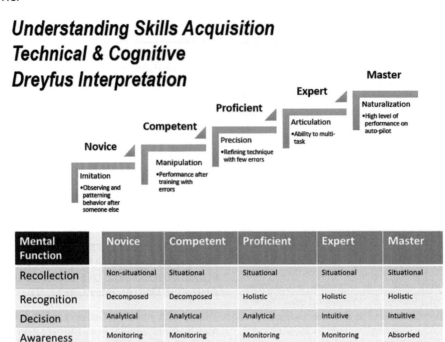

Fig. 2. Basic skills acquisition model based on Dreyfus interpretation. (*Courtesy of* Robert Sweet and Edward D. Verrier, MD, University of Washington, Seattle, WA.)

training. Let us leave "mastery" out of the current resident education discussion, because that might require wisdom, leadership, presence, charisma, or other nonsurgical skills and should be sustained over time, so therefore maybe only obtained by an elite few. Yet, most of us would hope that at the end of residency, our trainees are approaching a level of expertise rather than competency. *If a surgeon is going to operate on my mother or child when they finish training, I would prefer that she or he be an expert rather than simply being "competent".* The corollary concept to expertise then is the practical issue of autonomy: by the completion of training.[20,21] Right now in general surgery almost 90% of the trainees take an additional year of subspecialty or advanced fellowship training.[22] We in cardiothoracic surgery may be similarly approaching that percentage if we add in those going on to congenital, adult congenital, structural heart, mechanical circulatory assist, or transplantation fellowships in cardiothoracic surgery. Obviously, subspecialization may have advantages in the marketplace for young trainees, but an evolving concept is that many residents in training are not given the opportunity to become autonomous in either their decision-making (cognitive) or in the operating room (technical skills) at the end of their regular training. That then raises the additional issue of how we achieve expertise when we demand our resident be the jack of all trades (adult cardiac, thoracic, congenital, and critical care) but not necessarily the master of one.

Many countries around the world outside the United States have already separated the training in each of these areas. Finally, how do we then set the foundation standards for lifelong learning? Our specialty, especially adult cardiac surgery, is technology driven so technical advances have come rapidly (transcatheter approaches to valves and aortic disease, robotics, minimally invasive). Somewhat similarly thoracic surgery is being driven by translational research, which may dramatically change the horizons on how cancer (proton therapy, immunotherapy) will be treated in the future. We therefore all live in new multidisciplinary worlds devoid of the classic safe silos of knowledge, finance, politics, and identity such as medicine, radiology, and surgery. How do we then provide credible continuing medical education and ongoing credentialing as part of lifelong learning and expertise? Should those standards be exclusively left to societies and hospital or do we have responsibility as surgical educators to establish standards based on the science of adult learning, accurate assessment, formative feedback, faculty development and training, educational technology, and the new frontiers of surgical education?

NEW FRONTIERS IN SURGICAL EDUCATION

As we look forward at our educational paradigm there certainly seem to be some challenging frontiers in surgery. There probably will be no substitute for hands on, game day experiences in the operating room with live patients and well-trained surgical educators. But the challenges in the operating room are real: financial margins for the hospital almost cannot afford the time or distraction of education, outcomes and safety are increasing in importance while transparency of outcome data is real and analyzed, patient complexity and risk continues to increase, and subspecialization of providers make the basic surgical foundation even more challenging to establish. Even the ever changing impact of technology evolution means that what you learn today may be completely outdated tomorrow.

- Where then does simulation fit in? High-fidelity expensive simulators usually lie dormant yet simple low-fidelity simulators do not seem real. Is simulation best used to train for uncommon but potentially lethal events? Many buildings have been built by philanthropic interests, buildings created to use simulation for safety (like in the airline industry) but then remain empty without curriculum buy-in or ongoing commitment.[23,24]
- It is clear that traditionally we in medicine, and particularly in surgery, carry significant "implicit bias." We more likely than not still carry the stigmata of the "old boys" club. How do we better, proactively minimize gender, racial, age, leadership, or any other implicit bias?[25]
- Futurists say the virtual or augmented reality and artificial intelligence will drive our global economies for the next generation and we can see the investments that up and coming economies such as India and China are making in these arenas. Should not they also be part of our medical and surgical frontiers in education?[26,27]
- Why cannot we create a link between current imaging technology (computed tomographic scans, MRI, echocardiography) and computer science to create virtual or augmented reality environment that are more than games to be used in real time to visualize or teach complex 3-dimensional anatomy or pathology in surgery? This could then allow preparation, rehearsal, warm up, and thereby improve our educational environment and outcomes. Could not this also be used to improve technical skill preparation, performance, and assessment?[28]
- If we make the assumption that the triangle of knowledge moves from measurement to facts, to data, to information, to knowledge, and to wisdom (**Fig. 3**), it is clear we are moving from the current era of information (guidelines, levels of evidence) into the era of

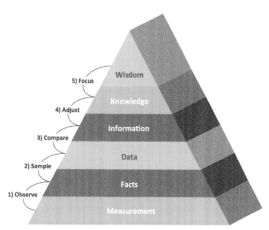

Fig. 3. DIKW knowledge pyramid.

knowledge. The concept of knowledge management systems are evolving and these will be driven by artificial intelligence (AI). Will not such resources as AI be increasingly used for clinical judgment and decision-making in medicine and should not we as surgeons be part of the design and implementation of such systems?[29]
- Anders Ericsson, the guru of deliberate practice and performance, has shown us that all elite performers (dancers, musicians, chess players, athletes, and even doctors) must practice, warm up, rehearse, and use coaches, yet most of those artists perform for pleasure and are not responsible for addressing human suffering.[30] Where should these habits be expected in surgery?
- Our current training algorithm in cardiothoracic surgery in the United States of having every resident complete intensive care, adult cardiac surgery, general thoracic surgery in order to sit for the Boards and then add on a year or two for congenital might need to be addressed if our goal is expertise in training rather than simple competency.

THE SURGEON AS EDUCATOR

The authors' goal with this issue is to provide an up to date "sentinel reference" for surgical educators but in addition be used to simulate academic opportunities for young surgeons interested in becoming true educators.[31] Being a good educator is simply not an art form you are born with or one you inherit simply by observation. Education is an academic discipline, which can provide a rich opportunity for young surgeons interested in significantly contributing to the next generation of surgeons in training or for personal career development in a unique but critically important way.

REFERENCES

1. Vaporciyan AA, Yang SC, Baker CJ, et al. Cardiothoracic surgery residency training: past, present and future. J Thorac Cardiovasc Surg 2013;146:759–67.
2. Verrier ED. The elite athlete the master surgeon. J Am Coll Surg 2017;224:225–35.
3. D'Cunha J, Schmitz CC, Maddaus MNA. Being an effective surgical educator. Thorac Surg Clin 2011; 21:359–68.
4. Flexner A. Medical education in the United States and Canada. Washington, DC: Science and Health Publications; 1910.
5. Cameron JL. William Halsted: our surgical heritage. Ann Surg 1997;225:445–58.
6. Grillo H. Edward D. Churchill and the "rectangular" surgical residency. Surgery 2004;136:947–53.
7. Sonnadara RR, Mui C, McQueen S, et al. Reflections on competency based education and training of surgical residents. J Surg Educ 2014;71:152–6.
8. Bell RH. Presidential address: why Johnny can't operate. Surgery 2009;146:533–41.
9. Robinson K. Out of our minds: learning to be creative. West Sussex (United Kingdom): Capstone; 2011.
10. Taylor DCM, Hamdy H. Adult learning theories: implications for learning and teaching in medical education: AMME guide No. 83. Med Teach 2013;35:11. E1561–1572.
11. Kolb DA. Experiential learning: experience as the source of learning and development. Englewood Cliffs (NJ): Prentice Hall; 1984.
12. Knowles MS. The modern practice of adult education. New York: Adult EducationCompany; 1980.
13. Davison S, Raison N, Khan MS, et al. Mental training in surgical education: a systematic review. Anz J Surg 2017;87:873–8.
14. Dearani J, Gold M, Leibovich BC, et al. The role of imaging, deliberate practice, structure, and improvisation in approaching surgical perfection. J Thorac Cardiovasc Surg 2017;154:1329–36.
15. Mokadam MA, Dardas TF, Hermsen JL, et al. Flipping the classroom: case-based learning, accountability, assessment, and feedback leads to a favorable change in culture. J Thorac Cardiovasc Surg 2017;153(4):987–96.e1.
16. Mayer RE. Multimedia learning. New York: Meyers; 2005.
17. Dreyfus SE, Hubert LA. Five Stage Model of Mental activities involved in directed skill acquisition. Washington, DC: Sorning Media; 1980.
18. Frank JR, Snell LS, Cate OT, et al. Competency-based medical education: theory to practice. Med Teach 2010;32(8):638–45.
19. Holmboe ES, Edgar L, Hamstra S. The Milestone Handbook (ACGME) (2016). Available at: milestones@acgme.org. Accessed January 2019.
20. Soper NJ, DaRosa DA. Presidential address: engendering operative autonomy in surgical training. Surgery 2014;156:745–51.
21. Sandhu G, Teman NR. Training autonomous surgeons: more time or faculty development? Ann Surg 2015;261:843–5.
22. Sorensen MJ. Surgical subspecialization: escape route for surgeons or added benefit for patients? J Grad Med Educ 2014;6(2):215–7.
23. Feins RH, Burkhart HM, Conte JV, et al. Simulation-based training in cardiac surgery. Ann Thorac Surg 2017;103:312–21.
24. Mokadam NA, Fann JI, Hicks GL, et al. Experience with the cardiac surgery simulation curriculum: results of the resident and faculty survey. Ann Thorac Surg 2017;103:322–8.
25. Banaji MR, Greenwald AG. Blindspot: hidden biases of good people. New York: Bantam Books; 2016.
26. Purdy M, Daugherty P. Artificial Intelligence is the future of growth. Available at: https://www.accenture.com/us-en/insight-artificial-intelligence-future-growth. Accessed January 2019.
27. Hall S, Takaahashi R. Augmented and virtual reality: the promise and perils of immersive technologies. Available at: https://www.weforum.org/agenda/2017/09/augmented-and-virtual-reality-will-change-how-we-create-and-consume-and-bring-new-risks/. Accessed January 2019.
28. Palter VN, Grantcharov TP. Individualized deliberate practice on a virtual reality simulator improves technical performance of surgical novices in the operating room: a randomized controlled trial. Ann Surg 2014;259(3):443–8.
29. Hashimoto DA, Rosman G, Rus D, et al. Artificial intelligence in surgery: promises and pitfalls. Ann Surg 2018;268(1):70–9.
30. Ericsson KA, Pool R. Peak: secrets from the new science of expertise. New York: Ericsson; 2016.
31. Klingensmith ME, Anderson KD. Educational scholarship as a route to academic promotion: a depiction of surgical education scholars. Am J Surg 2006;191:533–7.

How Does the Adult Surgeon Learn?

Kathleen Berfield, MD

KEYWORDS

• Surgical education • Adult learning • Resident education • Surgery resident

KEY POINTS

- Both the breadth of knowledge and range of technical skills that residents are now expected to master prior to graduation have grown exponentially.
- A unique challenge that sets surgical education apart from medical education is that surgery as a specialty requires not only the mastery of complex physiology, anatomy, and disease processes but also the ability to interpret and apply that knowledge in the operating room.
- To be effective educators, it is imperative to understand the theoretic foundation of how adults learn.

Halsted's[1] principles of surgical education (**Box 1**), which call for graded autonomy and the progressive transfer of patient care from the attending surgeon to the trainee, are the foundation on which surgical training has been built.[1,2] Although the apprenticeship model is still widely used and Halsted's principles remain the aim of surgical training, the landscape of surgical education has changed significantly. Both the breadth of knowledge and range of technical skills that residents are now expected to master prior to graduation have grown exponentially. Limits on work hours and changes in case volume and supervision requirements all add to the complexity of ensuring residents receive adequate training to become competent and capable surgeons.

A unique challenge that sets surgical education apart from medical education is that surgery as a specialty requires not only the mastery of complex physiology, anatomy, and disease processes but also the ability to interpret and apply that knowledge in the operating room. It is the interplay of knowledge, judgment, and technical skills that make a *surgeon*. Although attending surgeons are regularly called on to be educators, coaches,

and mentors to residents, few actually receive formal training on how to teach effectively. Furthermore, new pressures from society and hospital administration for better patient outcomes and satisfaction, productivity, and cost-effective care all make prioritizing education difficult. No single learning theory can fully capture the complexity of surgical education and training. To be effective educators, however, it is imperative to understand the theoretic foundation of how adults learn. The aim of this article is not to describe all adult learning theory but to introduce the reader to a few theories and concepts that can be integrated into day-to-day practice to help facilitate learning in surgical trainees.

Understanding how adults learn begins with understanding *andragogy*, which is defined as the "art and science of helping adults learn."[3] The andragogical model as described by Malcolm Knowles and colleagues[3], is composed of 6 assumptions and is believed a cornerstone of adult learning (**Box 2**). The andragogical model is meant to be flexible and Knowles' intention is that it can be adopted or adapted in whole or in part, befitting the learner and the circumstance.

Disclosure: The author has nothing to disclose.
Department of Surgery, Division of CT Surgery, University of Washington, UWMC, 1959 Northeast Pacific Street, Box 356310, Seattle, WA 98195, USA
E-mail address: berfield@uw.edu

Thorac Surg Clin 29 (2019) 233–238
https://doi.org/10.1016/j.thorsurg.2019.04.001

Box 1
Halsted's principles of surgical training

- The resident must have intense and repetitive opportunities to take care of surgical patients under the supervision of a skilled surgical teacher.
- The resident must acquire an understanding of the scientific basis of surgical disease.
- The resident must acquire skills in patient management and technical operations of increasing complexity with graded enhanced responsibility and independence.[1]

activities challenge the concept of being self-directing and create a psychological conflict for which the typical instinct is to escape or flee from the situation. Knowles posits that this may account for the high dropout rates in adult education. It is not difficult to see how residents' self-concept might be similarly challenged throughout training, whether it is being told they are not performing well in the operating room or failing to remember all the indications for a certain intervention. Thus, part of the challenge for surgical educators is to be aware of this problem and find ways to create learning experiences that build on rather than conflict with the self-concept of trainees.

THE NEED TO KNOW

Knowles states that adult learners "need to know why they should learn something."[3] When adults understand why they should learn something and how learning or not learning will have a positive or negative impact on them, they will invest more in the process of learning. Therefore, to ensure success in residents, it is imperative that they understand the benefit that learning will bring them. Fortunately, for much of surgical training, the concept of need to know is straightforward. Most residents in a cardiothoracic surgery residency understand the importance of knowing how to cannulate for bypass or to perform a thoracotomy. Part of the role of surgical educators, is to help residents become aware of the need to know such that they can discover for themselves where the gaps lie in their knowledge or technical skills.

THE LEARNERS' SELF-CONCEPT

In contrast to children, adults have a self-concept of themselves as being self-directing, capable, and responsible for their own lives. Once this self-concept has developed, adults then have a psychological need to be seen in this light and resist and resent situations that challenge this notion of self. Formal training or education

THE ROLE OF THE LEARNERS' EXPERIENCES

Another assumption of the Andragogical model holds that each adult accumulates a wide range of life experiences, which then influence how they approach learning and their own education. As such, the methods utilized to facilitate learning in residents require greater individualization of learning strategies and methods of teaching. Mental habits also form as a result of prior experiences, resulting in biases and presuppositions that may hinder new learning.[3] Mezirow's transformative learning theory also supports this assumption and states that "transformative learning is the process by which we internalize and interpret information based on our own experiences."[4,5] Mezirow goes on to state that transformation in learning takes place as a result of the learning process itself and is a social process. Both Knowles and Mezirow encourage the use of the learners' own experiences and encourage group discussion, simulation, and peer-based teaching to promote learning. As surgical educators, it is necessary to be cognizant of residents' experiences and how they have an impact on their training and how educators can capitalize on their prior experiences to guide and support their learning.

READINESS TO LEARN

Adults are ready to learn something when it becomes pertinent to their real-life situation. Implicit to readiness to learn is the importance of timing new learning experiences to coincide with developmental tasks that address the learning need at hand. For the authors' surgical trainees, the expectation of graded autonomy helps reinforce a sense of constant readiness. A resident need only look to the next most senior resident to understand what is expected and needs to be learned. For residents who struggle with this, Knowles states that readiness is inducible and can be

Box 2
Andragogical model

1. The need to know
2. The learners' self-concept
3. The role of the learners' experiences
4. Readiness to learn
5. Orientation to learning
6. Motivation

encouraged through exposure, simulation, and counseling.

ORIENTATION TO LEARNING

Adult learners are task centered or problem centered with respect to learning in comparison to children, who are subject centered. As such, adults' interest in learning is proportional to how much they perceive learning will help them perform tasks or manage problems that will be encountered. Moreover, learning occurs most effectively when it is presented in the context of application to real-life situations. Within the field of surgical education, simulation is the perfect tool to capitalize on this assumption and is discussed further in Phillip G. Rowse and Joseph A. Dearani's article, "Deliberate Practice and the Emerging Roles of Simulation in Thoracic Surgery," in this issue.

MOTIVATION

The last assumption is that adults find more motivation in internal factors, such as quality of life, job satisfaction, and self-esteem, than they do in external factors, such as promotions, higher salary, and recognition. Additional research has shown that all normal adults are internally motivated to continue growing and developing. The motivation to learn is further explained by Wlodowski,[6] who states that the motivation to learn is the sum of 4 factors: success, volition, value, and enjoyment. In other words, adults want to be successful learners, who can choose what they learn and find value and joy in what they are learning.[3,6]

A commonly held belief in the field of adult learning is that adults cannot be forced to learn. Rather, learning is a willful act on the part of the learner.[7] This concept of self-directed learning (SDL) or autonomous learning is central to andragogy (**Box 3**). Knowles described SDL as "a process in which individuals take the initiative, with or without the help of others, in diagnosing their learning needs, formulating goals, identifying human and material resources for learning, choosing and implementing appropriate learning strategies, and evaluating learning outcomes."[8] Although the concept of SDL is widely accepted in the field of adult learning research, there are 2 views of what SDL entails. The first view is that SDL is "self-teaching" whereby learners can control the style and manner in which they teach themselves. The second view is that the learner has "personal autonomy" in learning and assumes ownership of the goals and purposes of their learning.[9] Although these 2 views of SDL differ, they are not mutually exclusive. Grow[10] suggests that SDL is based on

---

> **Box 3**
> **Self-directed learning**
>
> SDL is a process in which individuals take the initiative, with or without the help of others, in diagnosing their learning needs, formulating goals, identifying human and material resources of learning, choosing and implementing appropriate learning strategies, and evaluating learning outcomes.[8]

the individual learner and the context of the learning at hand; as such, the role of the educator is to match styles with the trainee.[3,10]

PROCESSES OF LEARNING

The andragogical model is a process model (**Box 4**) rather than a content model, wherein rather than focusing on the transmission of information and skills from teacher to learner, the emphasis is placed on "providing procedures and resources for helping learners acquire information and skills."[3] In this model, educators' role is to facilitate learning rather than presenting learners with prefabricated learning plans or agendas. The concept underlying the process model of learning is to engage the learner in the learning experience.

Since andragogy was initially described, many new perspectives on adult learning have emerged that can be used to augment understanding of adult learning theory. A few concepts particularly relevant to surgical education are reflection, transformative learning, experiential learning, and the social context of learning.

Knowing-in-action and reflection-in-action, described by Schon,[11] are processes where the use of known mental schema enable the trainee to successfully perform certain tasks. Knowing-in-action is an automatic, reflexive response that allows a resident to efficiently perform a task on a daily basis. Reflection-in-action is the process of actively reflecting on the performance of those

---

> **Box 4**
> **Process model**
>
> - Prepare the learner
> - Establish a climate conducive to learning
> - Create a mechanism for mutual planning
> - Diagnose the needs for learning
> - Set objectives that satisfy these needs
> - Design the learning experience
> - Conduct the learning experience
> - Evaluate the outcomes and rediagnose needs

tasks, testing the associated mental schema, and then making changes to those schemata when necessary. Reflection-in-action allows for the fine tuning of skills and knowledge and ultimately results in personal and professional growth. The use of formal feedback and debriefing after cases is an example of using reflection in surgical training.

Transformative learning also calls on the use of reflection and is used to describe the learning process wherein new information is interpreted and filtered based on prior experiences; this is a common theme in adult learning theory. In this case, the transformation refers to the evolution of an existing way of thinking into something new based on what has been learned during the process and uses self-reflection to challenge a learner's assumptions and beliefs. Transformative learning can be promoted by encouraging discussion and group participation among residents and faculty.[4,5,7] Uses of regular morbidity and mortality conferences or case review conferences are examples where both reflection and transformative learning can and are utilized.

Experiential learning taps into the general preference of adults to learn through new experiences and problem solving. As described by Kolb,[12] experiential learning consists of 4 steps, which he refers to as the learning cycle:

1. Performing a task
2. Observation of and reflection on the learners' experience
3. Integration of new information into a new concept or paradigm
4. Testing and incorporating the new paradigm into the next task

Experiential learning can be used to design adult learning experiences and is essentially on-the-job training. The clinical years during medical school rely on experiential learning through the completion of core clinical rotations, and human resource development leaders frequently use experiential learning as a tool to improve the performance of both individuals and teams.

Situated learning theory highlights how the social context of learning influences how people learn. Not only is learning, therefore, the transformation of knowledge but also learning incorporates environmental, cultural, interpersonal, and social factors.[13–15] Three underlying assumptions of situated learning are as follows:

1. Learning and thinking are social activities.
2. Learning and thinking are structured by the tools available in specific situations
3. Thinking is influenced by the setting in which learning takes place.

In this model, learning is both explicit and implicit, such that the "hidden curriculum" or mixed messages from attendings can undermine even the best of learning experiences.[15] The implication of situational learning theory is that learning is influenced by the culture or "community of practice" and, therefore, surgical educators must be deliberate about modeling the behavior and actions they want their residents to emulate.

Mind-brain education science is an emerging field that integrates education, psychology, and neurobiology to better characterize and understand how people learn and is especially fitting for surgical education. Bloom and colleagues[16] propose that there are 3 domains of learning: cognitive, psychomotor, and affective, which separate the intellectual processes from the physical and emotional processes, respectively. Most learning experiences involve all 3 domains, and neurobiologists have demonstrated that when learning involves multiple domains it is more powerful and longer lasting.[17]

Learning results in structural and functional changes in neural networks in the brain as well as new neuron generation, and learning experiences are dynamic and subject to external factors that can be strengthened or weakened by elements of the learning experience itself or post hoc alterations.[18,19] These learning experiences must be reinforced to be maintained and improved on. It will come as no surprise that learning is influenced by emotions—positive feelings enhance learning and negative feelings hinder learning.[20] The reason behind this can be further explained with an understanding of neurobiology. Positive emotions during learning have been shown to trigger the release of neurotransmitters, including dopamine, which enhance the uptake of information.[21] Conversely, adrenaline is released during stressful learning, which distracts the learner from the experience at hand and shifts their attention to the fight or flight instinct, thereby inhibiting the uptake of information.[22] Sousa further describes a hierarchy in responses in which sensory data and emotional data override other stimuli and processes, such that sensory input that is perceived as a threat (being yelled at in an operating room, for example) also results in the release of adrenaline, which inhibits learning. The implication is that how a learner feels about a learning event influences the ability to learn from it. Friedlander and colleagues[23] have further identified 10 concepts that are key to memory formation and learning (**Box 5**).

Although the perfect timing of repetition is yet unknown, Friedlander and colleagues[23] report that repetition and revisiting the same topic from

> **Box 5**
> **Key concepts from the neurobiology of learning**
>
> - Repetition
> - Reward and reinforcement
> - Visualization
> - Active engagement
> - Stress
> - Fatigue
> - Multitasking
> - Individual learning styles
> - Active involvement
> - Revisiting information/concepts through multimedia/sensory processes

different perspectives are important and that repetition and redundancy act to strengthen neural pathways, making them more efficient offloading to lower-order pathways, thereby leaving higher-order pathways available for cognitive processing. Given these findings, the formal use of deliberate practice and simulation are invaluable tools to help facilitate learning, particularly for the more the technical aspects of surgery. Additionally, the use of defined curriculums, such as the thoracic surgical curriculum, which can be recycled throughout cardiothoracic surgery residency, can help reinforce learning through repetition.

The field of surgery continues to evolve and grow and with this change so too must the methods of educating surgical residents. So how do surgical educators apply their knowledge of andragogy and adult learning theory? First, the idea of SDL among residents must be leveraged. Just like Halsted's principles, the concept of autonomy is a key component of SDL. With the transition to competency-based training and the use of milestones to track residents' progress throughout training, now more than ever residents must be empowered to drive their own education processes and be responsible for their training. Residents should be actively involved in the creation of their educational curriculum and selection of their learning resources to ensure resident buy-in and engagement It also must be remembered that learning crosses domains and can be reinforced by not only physical and cognitive cues but also cultural and environmental cues. Finally, educators must not be married to one method of learning or teaching. Rather successful surgeon educators should strive to be flexible and tailor their methods to the needs of individual surgeons in training.

REFERENCES

1. Polavarapu HV, Kulaylat AN, Sun S, et al. 100 years of surgical education: the past, present, and future. Bull Am Coll Surg 2013;98(7):22–7.
2. Cameron JL. William Stewart Halsted: our surgical heritage. Ann Surg 1997;225(5):445–58.
3. Knowles MS, Holton EF, Swanson RA. The adult learner: the definitive classic in adult education and human resource development. 8th edition. Houston (TX): Gulf; 2015.
4. Mezirow J. Transformative dimensions of adult learning. San Francisco (CA): Jossey-Bass; 1991.
5. Rashid P. Surgical education and adult learning: integrating theory into practice. F1000Res 2017;6:143.
6. Wlodowski RJ. Enhancing adult motivation to learn. San Francisco (CA): Jossey-Bass; 1985.
7. Mackeracher DMG. Making sense of adult learning 2nd edition. Buffalo (NY): University of Toronto Press; 2004.
8. Knowles M. Self-directed learning: a guide for learners and teachers. New York: Associated Press; 1975. p. 18.
9. Candy PC. Self direction for lifelong learning. San Francisco (CA): Jossey-Bass; 1991.
10. Grow GO. Teaching learners to be self directed. Adult Educ Q 1991;41:125–49.
11. Schon DA. Educating the reflective practitioner. San Francisco (CA): Jossey-Bass; 1987.
12. Kolb DA. Experiential learning: experience as the source of learning and development. Englewood-Cliffs (NJ): Prentice-Hall; 1984.
13. Taylor DCM, Hamdy H. Adult learning theories: Implications for learning and teaching in medical education: AMEE Guide No. 83. Med Teach 2013;35(11):e1561–72.
14. Durning SJ, Artino AR. Situativity theory: a perspective on how participants and the environment can interact: AMEE Guide no. 52. Med Teach 2011;33:188–99.
15. Schumacher D, Englander R, Carraccio C. Developing the master learner: applying learning theory to the learner, the teacher and the learning environment. Academic Medicine 2013;88(11):1635–45.
16. Bloom BS, ENgelhart MD, Furst EJ, et al. "Taxonomy of educational objectives." The classification of educational goals: Handbook 1: cognitive domain. New York: Longmans, Green; 1956.
17. Mahan JD, Stein DS. Teaching adults — best practices that leverage the emerging understanding of the neurobiology of learning. Curr Probl Pediatr Adolesc Health Care 2014;44(6):141–9.
18. Glick M. The instructional leader and the brain: using neuroscience to inform practice. Thousand Oaks (CA): Sage; 2011.
19. Uncapher MR, Rugg MD. Selecting for memory? the influence of selective attention on the mnemonic binding of contextual information. J Neurosci 2009; 29(25):8270–9.

20. Zull JE. The art of changing the brain: enriching the practice of teaching by exploring the biology of learning. Sterling (VA): Stylus Publishing; 2002.

21. Tokuhama-Espinosa T. Mind, brain, and education science : a comprehensive guide to the new brain-based teaching. 1st edition. New York: W.W. Norton; 2011.

22. Wolf P. The role of meaning and emotion and learning. New Directions for Adult and Continuing Education 2006;100:35–41.

23. Friedlander MJ, Linda Andrews MD, Armstrong EG, et al. What can medical education learn from the neurobiology of learning? Acad Med 2011;86: 415–20.

Obtaining Meaningful Assessment in Thoracic Surgery Education

Amy L. Holmstrom, MD[a], Shari L. Meyerson, MD, MEd[b],*

KEYWORDS

- Surgical assessment • Surgical education • Entrustable professional activities
- Competency-based medical education

KEY POINTS

- Traditional mechanisms of assessment of the surgical trainee include standardized multiple-choice examinations, oral examinations, and meticulous case logs.
- Assessment of the surgical trainee is evolving toward a competency-based approach that includes in vivo observations of clinical and operative clinical encounters in addition to standardized simulation-based assessment tools.
- Transition to competency-based assessments will emphasize holistic evaluations that are learner centered and are independent of time.

INTRODUCTION

Certification boards, such as the American Board of Thoracic Surgery (ABTS), have as one of their primary goals protecting the public by ensuring that surgeons are safe and competent to practice independently. Over the past number of decades, however, the training itself has changed. The amount of information residents needs to learn grows every year as the field expands. External pressures on surgeons, such as increased public scrutiny of outcomes, and financial pressure to use operating time efficiently and increase case volumes have resulted in less time for teaching and decreased resident autonomy.[1-4] And finally, resident work hour rules control the amount of time residents can spend learning in the hospital.[5] There is growing concern that residents are not prepared for practice.[6] Thoracic residents themselves identified several operative procedures where they believed they needed more instruction or lacked confidence, including minimally invasive cardiac and esophageal operations, all types of robotic operations, endovascular operations, and operations for congenital cardiac conditions.[7] These challenges to training make accurate assessment of competency even more crucial than it has been in the past. Although these challenges may seem insurmountable, a re-evaluation of scope of residency with simultaneous adjustments to assessment methods may allow programs to better define what is expected of a competent thoracic surgeon at the end of their residency training.

Competency often has been assessed using a siloed approach, including evaluations of fund of knowledge, clinical judgment, and technical skill. Assessment of these domains of practice by the training program faculty along with documentation of experience based on case logs and passage of a predetermined amount of time (24 months for a 2-year fellowship or 72 months for a 6-year

Disclosure Statement: The authors have nothing to disclose.
[a] Department of Surgery, Northwestern University Feinberg School of Medicine, 676 North Saint Clair Street, Suite 2320, Chicago, IL 60611, USA; [b] Department of Surgery, University of Kentucky, 740 South Limestone, Suite A301, Lexington, KY 40536, USA
* Corresponding author.
E-mail address: shari.meyerson@uky.edu

Thorac Surg Clin 29 (2019) 239–247
https://doi.org/10.1016/j.thorsurg.2019.03.002

integrated program) are required for board eligibility. The ABTS then administers 2 summative evaluations, the qualifying and certifying examinations, which a graduate must pass before being declared board certified. Over the past decade, the idea of competency-based education has begun to influence changes in medical educational curricula. Competency-based medical education aims to take a learner-centered, outcomes-based approach to training physicians instead of the traditional, siloed approach. As defined by Frank and colleagues,[8] competency-based medical education de-emphasizes time and focuses on abilities of trainees, organized around disease-specific and procedure-specific competencies. As competency-based medical education enters the mainstream of the medical education world, it becomes vitally important to have robust and accurate assessment tools to determine competency.

This article begins by discussing the traditional domains that define trainee competence and associated methods of assessment. The role of competency-based medical education then is explored, including the integration and development of competency-based assessment tools and the potential future implications for surgical trainees.

AIMS OF ASSESSMENT

In order to have a meaningful discussion of assessment, it is important to first consider the aims of assessment. If the goal of surgical training is to create a competent surgeon, then competence itself must be defined. A competent surgeon can safely diagnose a patient with a surgical problem, perform the necessary operative intervention (or know when nonoperative management is a safe and preferred treatment), and care for the patient in both the preoperative and postoperative phases. A competent surgeon must have the necessary knowledge, clinical judgment, and technical abilities to carry out all of these aspects of patient care safely and accurately.

SILOED APPROACH TO ASSESSMENT

The most commonly used assessment mechanisms address 1 or more domain of clinical competence. Broadly, they can be grouped into the 3 main categories, listed previously: assessment of fund of knowledge, clinical judgment, and technical skills.

Fund of Knowledge

Fund of knowledge is the domain of competence that is tested most easily in a standardized fashion.

Trainees are expected to understand the relevant anatomy, pathophysiology, evaluation, and management of all disease processes commonly and uncommonly seen in thoracic surgery. The foundations of this knowledge are learned in medical school. During residency, trainees both expand their knowledge base and become more focused, developing in-depth knowledge of treatment options, operative procedures, and care of cardiac and thoracic patients.

Formal assessment of fund of knowledge traditionally has been performed using standardized, multiple-choice examinations. Multiple-choice examinations are a component of almost every aspect of acceptance into or advancement within medical educational curricula. There are several standardized examinations that all medical trainees must take prior to advancing to a surgical residency (United States Medical Licensing Examination), which then give way to annual in-training examinations. Other curricula embedded within surgical training, such as Advanced Trauma Life Support, Advanced Cardiac Life Support, and Fundamentals of Laparoscopic Surgery, all have a written component that is a multiple-choice examination. The benefits of this ubiquitous form of assessment are the ability to test many trainees simultaneously, the ease of administration and evaluation, and the cost effectiveness. It also is an efficient and reliable way to test a large breadth of knowledge across a variety of clinical situations.[9]

When combined with other forms of assessment, multiple-choice examinations are a useful assessment tool; however, they have low validity when used alone.[9] Limitations are evident for the surgical trainee because there is no way to test technical skill or ability to integrate real-time clinical information to make decisions. This corresponds to the strongest criticism of multiple-choice examinations, which is the encouragement of rote memorization instead of true understanding of material tested.

Clinical Judgment

The practical application and integration of knowledge with real-time clinical data to make patient care decisions can broadly be described as a trainee's clinical judgment. A competent thoracic surgeon should be able to properly evaluate, diagnose, and suggest a management plan for a patient with a potential surgical problem. Clinical judgment is also critically important for intraoperative decisions, which require the understanding of a disease process and potential complications to make choices in the operating room (eg, choice of pleurodesis mechanism or conversion from a minimally invasive to open approach).

Postoperative care requires the understanding of the typical postoperative course in addition to daily monitoring of the clinical examination and data for the development of potential complications. Good clinical judgment involves synthesis of fund of knowledge with data obtained in clinical settings as well as a nuanced understanding of the risks and benefits of each decision in the context of an individual patient.

Informal assessment of clinical judgment is one of the hallmarks of all surgical training, with daily interactions with supervising clinicians (senior residents, fellows, and attendings) allowing for ongoing assessment of a trainee's judgment. These informal daily assessments are formalized at the end of each rotation when faculty complete a standardized end-of-rotation evaluation. This usually is a computerized form filled out after the rotation is completed containing rating scales for various domains as well as an opportunity to provide qualitative feedback. End-of-rotation evaluations rarely provide useful evaluation or feedback for several reasons. They are filled out after completion of the rotation, sometimes weeks to months later, and faculty rarely remember any specific details about a resident's performance. Although the global rating and impression may be accurate, feedback given is often less than useful because it contains no specific ways for the resident to improve, often including phrases, such as "good job," "skills appropriate for level of training," or "needs to read more." For a more detailed discussion of formative feedback, see Leah M. Backhus and colleagues' the article, "Unconscious Bias: Addressing the Hidden Impact on Surgical Education," in this issue.

End-of-rotation evaluations have a significant risk of bias and lack of reproducibility.[10] Depending on the most recent interactions between the rater and the trainee, the evaluation may be impacted either positively or negatively regardless of prior performances, a form of bias known as the recency effect.[11,12] Similarly, negative thoughts or outcomes have a more lasting impact than do equivalent neutral or positive events, leading to greater negative impact on the overall evaluation, known as negativity bias. The halo effect is when positive attributes, such as professionalism, reliability, or simply a likable personality, are extrapolated to the remainder of a trainee's evaluation, leading to unwarranted positive or high marks across all components of the assessment. Surgical teams are highly dependent on teamwork but this can also create evaluation bias. A strong resident can make the other members of the team look better than they actually are. Conversely, a struggling resident can have a negative impact on a team's performance,

decreasing evaluation scores for those around them through group attribution error. For a more in-depth discussion of the effect of bias on surgical education, see Leah M. Backhus and colleagues' article, "Unconscious Bias: Addressing the Hidden Impact on Surgical Education," in this issue.

The structured summative assessment of clinical judgment occurs in the ABTS certification examination. This oral examination aims to test a trainee's clinical judgment and reasoning by evaluating responses to clinical scenarios. Examiners have the flexibility to change the clinical scenario to test the examinee's ability to integrate clinical information and make management decisions. This also allows an examiner to probe the examinee's depth of knowledge as well as assess adaptability and problem-solving ability. Another perceived strength of the oral examination format is the direct evaluation of professionalism, communication, and interpersonal skills.

The limitations of this examination are related to objectivity and standardization. Some of these limitations are born from the strengths of the examination, such as the flexibility allowed to the examiners, which makes standardization challenging. Evaluation of performance also is up to the examiners, which is subject to bias and mandates careful examiner training. There has been concern that some examinees might be disadvantaged due to performance anxiety.[13,14] Other investigators note the value of evaluating trainees in a stressful format because this replicates real-life clinical scenarios in which competent surgeons must be able to integrate information as they receive it and perform under stress. Proponents of this format argue, therefore, that oral examinations should remain a requisite component of the assessment of surgeons.[14–16]

Technical Proficiency

Finally, the technical ability of the trainee is an important factor that must be assessed prior to determining competence. There are many elements of surgical dexterity including but not limited to tissue handling, understanding and development of tissue planes, facile instrument use, economy of motion, use of tension and countertension, ability to obtain adequate exposure, and tying sutures under the correct tension with respect to tissue integrity.[17] The widespread use of minimally invasive techniques, such as laparoscopy, thoracoscopy, endoscopy, and robotic-assisted surgery, has added an additional layer of complexity to the technical assessment of trainees. Trainees develop their technical ability at different paces but, at a minimum, require broad and frequent exposure to technical procedures and operations to improve and advance their technical abilities.

Accurate methods of assessment of technical proficiency have been elusive. The only standardized skills assessment required to take the ABTS qualifying and certifying examinations is the Fundamentals of Laparoscopic Surgery. This skills assessment is performed on a box trainer, where examinees must complete 5 specific tasks with explicit criteria in a given time limit. These tasks are believed basic and essential laparoscopic skills and include peg transfer, precision cutting, endoloop, and suture with intracorporeal and extracorporeal knot tying.

As with other domains of trainee competence, assessment is documented in end-of-rotation evaluations, which can be subject to bias and poor reliability. The other required approach used to measure a trainee's technical skills, case logs, is really a surrogate for experience. There currently are few to no data to support the use of a specific number of cases to determine competence. A recent study indicated that it may take high numbers of performance of a single operation to develop a reproducible level of meaningful autonomy.[18] The investigators determined that a simple procedure like a laparoscopic appendectomy required at least 25 cases to reach meaningful autonomy reproducibly. Complex cases, such as partial colectomy, required up to 60 cases. The implications of this work for thoracic surgery where a truly complex procedure, such as esophagectomy, may be performed by a graduate who did only the minimum of 10 cases in training are interesting. One critical variable not measured in the case log is how much of the operation the resident actually performed and with what degree of autonomy. The ABTS requires a resident to perform those technical manipulations that constitute the essential parts of the procedure as well as are substantially involved in the preoperative and postoperative care of the patient in order to log a case. When surveyed, thoracic residents reported that only 70% to 75% of the cases they logged actually met this criteria, so their actual operative experience may be even less.[19] Residents also reported that only 2 common cardiac operations were performed routinely by graduating residents as the operative surgeon (coronary artery bypass grafting and aortic valve replacement).

USING COMPETENCY-BASED ASSESSMENTS TO ADDRESS SHORTCOMINGS OF THE SILOED APPROACH

It is evident that a competent surgeon utilizes knowledge, clinical judgment, and technical skills to safely and effectively care for patients. These skills are used simultaneously and fluidly during a patient encounter. Having an excellent fund of knowledge alone does not necessarily translate to competency in a clinical setting, and a trainee with excellent innate judgment can be limited by a poor fund of knowledge. Although technical skills are considered paramount in the actual performance of surgery, an operation cannot be progressed through without knowledge and clinical judgment. Knowledge helps a surgeon to identify and protect vital structures during an operation. Clinical judgment allows a surgeon to recognize when the operative plan needs to change.

Beyond the shortcomings of siloed assessments discussed previously, tools that evaluate skills separately are inherently limited in evaluating cumulative competence. The overall aim of assessment should be to evaluate the competency of a surgeon in training. Competency-based assessment tools aim to flip the traditional assessment paradigm. Rather than assess each component of competence separately, these methods aim to perform more complete, comprehensive evaluations of competency during a clinical encounter. Some competency-based assessments have already been integrated into training programs. Other novel attempts at comprehensive, competency-based assessment tools are still in development or are used as part of pilot programs or studies.

Milestones

The initial approach to competency-based medical education was spearheaded by the Accreditation Council for Graduate Medical Education (ACGME) with development of specialty-specific milestones. Milestones are designed to describe the progression from novice learner to competent surgeon in the set of 6 domains defined by the ACGME: medical knowledge, patient care, interpersonal and communication skills, professionalism, practice-based learning, and systems-based practice. Each milestone is a 5-step ladder with a series of examples of skills and behaviors that characterize each step. Trainees are expected to reach at least level 4 by the time of graduation in each of the milestones. The number of milestones varies widely between specialties, depending on the level of detail selected during development. The Thoracic Surgery Milestones were developed by a committee of thoracic surgeons under ACGME guidance in 2014 and consist of 26 separate milestones. A majority of the milestones are in the medical knowledge and patient care domains, which the committee chose to subdivide based on the major disease processes seen by thoracic surgeons, such as ischemic heart disease, lung and airway, and critical care.[20] Each training program has a Clinical Competency Committee composed of faculty who review the end-of-rotation evaluations and other forms of assessment to determine where a trainee falls on each milestone. Several aspects of milestones have proved useful. For the first time, they provided estimates of what a resident should be able to do at various levels of training, formally differentiating between simple and complex activities and behaviors. This creates a yardstick that can be used to determine if a resident is falling behind their peers to allow early remediation. Another useful aspect of the milestones is resident self-assessment, which allows for introspection on progression to competency during training and allows comparison to the faculty perception of progression. This helps the resident target self-study or deliberate practice in weak areas of knowledge or skills identified on the milestones. Many clinical competency committees, however, have struggled to assign meaningful milestones. This struggle is related to the lack of detail in most end-of-rotation evaluations, failure to observe or evaluate the specific types of behaviors noted in the milestones, or inadequate assessment tools.[21]

Assessment by Direct Observation

Competency-based assessment is best performed by real-time direct observation of resident performance. Given that much of the learning experience occurs during residents' day-to-day clinical activities, it is both convenient and cost effective to assess trainees by direct observation of these activities. These assessments also can act as formative feedback, allowing residents to correct their actions prior to the next patient encounter or operation rather than waiting until the end of the rotation. Observation and individual assessment of specific episodes of operative and clinical performance by faculty members only recently have become required for general surgery board eligibility but have not yet been adopted by the ABTS. The number of direct observation assessments required for general surgery residents currently is set at 12 assessments over 5 years, likely not adequate to truly estimate performance. One study showed that completion of 20 trainee observation assessments per year is sufficient to demonstrate a stable estimate of operative performance.[22] That translates to 40 assessments for a traditional 2-year thoracic fellowship and 120 assessments for a 6-year integrated thoracic surgery training program. The same study showed that

differences in the stringency of raters accounted for 3 times more variation in score than did the actual operative performance of the trainee.[22] This rater effect can be addressed by having at least 10 different raters per trainee per year to control for this variability although, in the often smaller thoracic faculty, it can be challenging to find that many raters compared with a larger general surgery faculty.[23] The main advantage of these real-time assessments is that they are performed immediately after the event, limiting recall biases. The value of direct observation performance assessments is diminished if there is a delay in time prior to completion of the form. After 3 days, the detail and clarity of the performance are lacking and it is suggested that assessments completed after this time should be discounted.[24] The main limitation of direct observation assessments is the administrative burden they create for both the trainee and the attending. Immediate evaluation is strongly encouraged, but this requires trainee ownership and faculty investment. Decreased trainee autonomy, a pervasive concern in current surgical training, also has an impact on observational assessments by limiting trainee opportunities to demonstrate their abilities. Direct observation assessments in the clinical setting currently are underutilized and undervalued as potential sources of significant trainee feedback and assessment.

Assessment of Surgical Skills in the Simulation Setting

As discussed previously, the only skills assessment required for ABTS board eligibility is the Fundamentals of Laparoscopic Surgery certification. Nonetheless, many training programs incorporate some form of skills assessment as a means of feedback to the trainee and to assess trainee progression. There are several validated technical skills assessment tools that have been developed, one of which is the Objective Structured Assessment of Technical Skills (OSATS). OSATS involves the performance of a series of standardized surgical tasks under the observation of a trained evaluator.[17,25] Performance is scored using a task-specific checklist in addition to a global rating form. Programs may choose to require trainees to pass procedure-specific verifications of proficiency prior to performance in a real clinical scenario. Trainees who fail a given task are mandated to remediate and retest until proficiency is attained. This is concordant with a competency-based curriculum because it focuses on the individual learner, and progress is independent of time. There are validated assessment tools available specifically designed for thoracic surgery procedures although they are not used routinely outside of the experimental setting. There are multiple tools that can be used for rating anatomic lung dissection based on the OSATS framework.[26–29] A validated assessment tool also exists for coronary artery anastomosis, which has been used not only for training but also as the assessment tool of the popular Top Gun competition run by the Society of Thoracic Surgeons annually.[30,31] Another tool available in the literature is used to assess cardiopulmonary bypass management, including crisis management.[32] These validated skills assessments are a method of ensuring all surgical trainees are proficient at basic and essential surgical skills.[33]

As technology advances, simulation for assessment will be extended to more complex skills and full procedures. There are now simulators that can replicate aortic cannulation complete with bleeding and virtual reality simulators, which allow trainees to practice video-assisted thoracoscopic surgery for anatomic lobectomy. Simulation for assessment allows the assessors to control the situation unlike in an actual patient. Complications can be planned and error management taught and evaluated. Some simulation settings also help eliminate bias by blinding the raters to the trainee's identity. Additionally, using simulation allows for even the most novice individual to attempt surgery with no inherent risk. The main limitation of simulation for assessment is the current state of technology. Current simulated surgery is not entirely realistic and has limited ability to mimic true clinical complications. As technology advances, especially virtual reality, which allows for nearly unlimited variation in clinical scenarios and anatomy, this will likely become less of a limitation.

Assessment of Surgical Skills in the Operating Room

The most commonly used scale for describing resident skills in the operating room is the Zwisch scale (**Table 1**).[34,35] This scale was named after its creator, Dr Joseph Zwischenberger, a thoracic surgeon who developed this language to assist his residents in achieving operative independence within constraints of a 2-year cardiothoracic surgery program.[34] The scale has 4 steps, starting at "show and tell," where the resident is an observer and assistant, and culminating at "supervision only," where the resident performs the procedure with only supervision from the attending, who acts to ensure the safety of the patient. The top 2 steps of this scale have been defined as meaningful autonomy, where the resident is

Table 1 The Zwisch scale of operative autonomy	
Zwisch Scale Rating	**Behavior**
Show and tell	Trainee: first assists Attending: performs >50% of critical portions of the operation, narrates the key concepts, skills, and anatomy of the case
Active help	Trainee: shifts between surgeon and first assist Attending: leads >50% of the operation, optimizes exposure, coaches regarding next steps and key technical points
Passive help	Trainee: can set up each step of the entire operation and recognizes critical transition points Attending: follows the lead of the trainee >50% of the operation, coaches for technical skills refinement
Supervision only	Trainee: can recover from most errors, knows when to seek advice/help Attending: acts as assistant or observes the trainee working with a junior assistant, largely provides no unsolicited advice

directing the flow of the operation. This scale has now been used in multiple smartphone-based applications: Zwisch Me (thoracic surgery), System for Improving and Measuring Procedural Learning (general surgery), and myTIPreport (obstetrics and gynecology). Faculty can enter their assessment of autonomy and performance at the end of a case as well as provide brief formative feedback to facilitate resident improvement. These apps have been shown to be a feasible, reliable, and valid method of operative performance assessment.[36] The combination of summative and formative assessment in near real time is one of the particular strengths of this assessment tool. The main limitation of these apps is the reliance on trainee and faculty buy-in to perform these assessments in a timely manner. Review of resident autonomy in relation to their level of training can highlight those who are not receiving expected autonomy and allow investigation into causes and help structure remediation plans. With frequent use at the program level, the Zwisch scale also may help identify faculty who consistently grant autonomy discordant with training level and/or who fail to provide feedback altogether. The Zwisch scale deployed as a smartphone-based application is a promising development toward achieving more frequent operative assessments and improving the value they provide to the trainee and the program about its trainees' progress toward competency.

Entrustable Professional Activities

The biggest struggle with assigning milestones to measure progress along the ACGME domains is that it can be difficult to isolate the domains from each other to evaluate them separately. A single clinical event, such as transitioning the care of a service of patients to the night shift, contains components of multiple milestones. Transitions of care are squarely in the domain of systems-based practice and initially seem straightforward to evaluate. If a resident fails to sign out that a postoperative cardiac patient is actively bleeding, however, it can be hard to tease out if the resident (1) did not know that was important to sign out, (2) did not know how much bleeding would be concerning, or (3) had not communicated with the nurse caring for that patient or any of numerous other potential reasons. These issues could fall under anything from medical knowledge to communication skills.

The next generation of competency-based assessment is shifting to entrustable professional activities (EPAs). This concept was developed by Olle ten Cate,[37] who postulated that it was more intuitive to assess whether or not trainees could perform the usual activities of clinical practice rather than trying to make clinical practice fit into the ACGME-defined domains. The scale used for EPAs is based on the amount of supervision the attending believes the resident requires to perform an activity and ranges from observation only to supervise others.

General surgery is piloting an EPA program for 5 core EPAs—evaluate and manage a patient presenting with right lower quadrant pain, gallbladder disease, inguinal hernia, and blunt or penetrating trauma, and provide surgical consultation. Evaluators are asked to rate the level of supervision to which they would entrust the trainee if faced with the same EPA in the future. Rather than evaluating a single event, EPAs are a cumulative evaluation where the level of trust granted is based not only on the event just observed but also on the history of prior similar encounters. This is a structured way to codify the decisions teaching faculty make every day.

Entrustment decisions cut across multiple core competencies encompassing not only knowledge and patient care but also professionalism, communication, and interpersonal skills. The biggest challenge of the EPA approach is the sheer number of professional activities most surgeons perform on a daily basis. It would be impossible to have multiple evaluations of every single activity and disease process that graduates are expected to be able to handle. There is work ahead to define what are the key EPAs that would be representative of the skills trainees need to learn. Although it remains a significant challenge, EPAs offer a potential avenue for more accurate assessment of a trainee's workplace performance and competence, especially with increasing evaluations of the same EPA by varying faculty. As with other performance evaluation tools, EPA evaluations take commitment/buy-in from the trainee and the faculty/evaluators.

Variable Training Time

Full implementation of competency-based medical education and assessment eventually may lead to a change in one of the fundamental underpinnings of surgical training: standardized training duration. It is well known that individuals learn at different paces; however, the inclusion of a time criteria in the requirements for board-eligibility defines the time spent training as an aspect of competence. It certainly takes time to become competent; but, because that time varies between residents, there needs to be a de-emphasis on arbitrary time periods and more emphasis on progression to competence. If a training program is able to give frequent, comprehensive assessments with feedback, individuals will have the ability to target specific areas for dedicated study and deliberate practice. This type of approach may result in early completion of training for some, but the more important and overarching goal will be for every graduate to finish training as a competent and confident surgeon regardless of the duration of training.

The orthopedic surgery residency program at the University of Toronto in Canada piloted a competency-based program in 2009 and then fully adopted a refined version in 2013 to 2014. The 8-year outcomes of this program were recently published and showed promising results.[38] The curriculum consisted of modules with specific competencies to be attained by completion of the module. Trainees had a minimum of 3 face-to-face meetings with the module supervisor to discuss learning objectives and assessments related to the module, assess progress, and perform a final assessment. Trainees progressing appropriately at the midmodule assessment would complete the module if competency was achieved at the final assessment, whereas others would formulate a learning plan and determine if additional time is needed for successful completion of the module. The trainees were given a teaching package composed of documents, training videos, and educational media for each module, allowing for self-directed study. Overall competency at the end of each module was assessed in a multimodal fashion including an oral and/or written examination, direct observations, and EPAs; 8 of the 14 residents in the pilot program completed their training in 4 years instead of the traditional 5-year time frame. One of the largest challenges faced was faculty development and increased investment in evaluating residents. Overall, the competency-based curriculum was independent of time, was learner centered, empowered residents, and established a more explicit attestation of competence that resulted in expeditious progression to competence for some trainees.

Time-independent learning also creates challenges related to case and disease process availability. If multiple residents were struggling with the same module, there may not be enough patient care opportunities. Conversely, this paradigm of training also may lead to residents progressing quickly through some modules. In the United States training system, in particular, hospitals rely on residents to care for patients. If all residents in a program have reached competency in a disease like empyema or straightforward aortic valve replacement, it will require a major investment from hospital systems to provide the care for those patients previously managed by residents. The successful implementation of a competency-based program by the University of Toronto is a model for other programs that may desire to move from a conventional time-based program to one based on competency.

SUMMARY

Meaningful assessment of the surgical trainee is evolving toward a multimodal, competency-based approach that forms a holistic evaluation of the trainee as a competent surgeon. The shift toward competency-based education has led to a need to assess the progression to competence through novel assessment tools and strategies. The key to successful assessment rests in a shift from classic end-of-rotation evaluations to frequent direct observation of clinical events with real-time evaluation and feedback. Programs must emphasize and mandate faculty educator training because it remains a crucial component of resident assessment. The ideal resident assessment will begin in the simulation setting to ensure basic skills. It will continue to the clinical setting with daily evaluations of clinical encounters perhaps using EPAs and measures of operative performance and autonomy to determine competency. Incorporating resident assessment into the daily workflow of faculty via simple smartphone-based applications is a necessary step toward achieving more frequent evaluations. Early and frequent assessment allows for targeted educational assistance for some and expeditious progression to competence for others. The overall result is a benefit to society and to the trainees, ensuring competence for all at completion of training and potentially reducing the time spent training for those who meet competency standards precociously.

REFERENCES

1. Hashimoto DA, Bynum WE 4th, Lillemoe KD, et al. See more, do more, teach more: surgical resident autonomy and the transition to independent practice. Acad Med 2016;91(6):757–60.
2. Guan J, Karsy M, Brock AA, et al. Overlapping surgery: a review of the controversy, the evidence, and future directions. Neurosurgery 2017;64(CN_suppl_1):110–3.
3. Coleman JJ, Esposito TJ, Rozycki GS, et al. Early subspecialization and perceived competence in surgical training: are residents ready? J Am Coll Surg 2013;216(4):764–71 [discussion: 771–3].
4. Patel M, Bhullar JS, Subhas G, et al. Present status of autonomy in surgical residency–a program director's perspective. Am Surg 2015;81(8): 786–90.
5. Borman KR, Jones AT, Shea JA. Duty hours, quality of care, and patient safety: general surgery resident perceptions. J Am Coll Surg 2012;215(1):70–7 [discussion: 77–9].
6. Mattar SG, Alseidi AA, Jones DB, et al. General surgery residency inadequately prepares trainees for fellowship: results of a survey of fellowship program directors. Ann Surg 2013;258(3):440–9.
7. Chu D, Vaporciyan AA, Iannettoni MD, et al. Are there gaps in current thoracic surgery residency training programs? Ann Thorac Surg 2016;101(6): 2350–5.

8. Frank JR, Mungroo R, Ahmad Y, et al. Toward a definition of competency-based education in medicine: a systematic review of published definitions. Med Teach 2010;32(8):631–7.

9. Moss E. Multiple choice questions: their value as an assessment tool. Curr Opin Anaesthesiol 2001; 14(6):661–6.

10. Yeates P, O'Neill P, Mann K, et al. Seeing the same thing differently: mechanisms that contribute to assessor differences in directly-observed performance assessments. Adv Health Sci Educ Theory Pract 2013;18(3):325–41.

11. Yeates P, O'Neill P, Mann K, et al. 'You're certainly relatively competent': assessor bias due to recent experiences. Med Educ 2013;47(9):910–22.

12. Yeates P, Cardell J, Byrne G, et al. Relatively speaking: contrast effects influence assessors' scores and narrative feedback. Med Educ 2015; 49(9):909–19.

13. Vergis A, Hardy K. Cognitive and technical skill assessment in surgical education: a changing horizon. Indian J Surg 2017;79(2):153–7.

14. Iqbal IZ, Naqvi S, Abeysundara L, et al. The value of oral assessments: a review. Ann R Coll Surg Engl 2010;92(Suppl):1–6.

15. Lunz ME, Bashook PG. Relationship between candidate communication ability and oral certification examination scores. Med Educ 2008;42(12):1227–33.

16. Epstein RM. Assessment in medical education. N Engl J Med 2007;356(4):387–96.

17. Martin JA, Regehr G, Reznick R, et al. Objective structured assessment of technical skill (OSATS) for surgical residents. Br J Surg 1997;84(2):273–8.

18. Stride HP, George BC, Williams RG, et al. Relationship of procedural numbers with meaningful procedural autonomy in general surgery residents. Surgery 2018;163(3):488–94.

19. Robich MP, Flagg A, LaPar DJ, et al. Understanding why residents may inaccurately log their role in operations: a look at the 2013 in-training examination survey. Ann Thorac Surg 2016;101(1):323–8.

20. The thoracic surgery milestone project. J Grad Med Educ 2014;6(1 Suppl 1):332–54.

21. Conforti LN, Yaghmour NA, Hamstra SJ, et al. The effect and use of milestones in the assessment of neurological surgery residents and residency programs. J Surg Ed 2018;75(1):147–55.

22. Williams RG, Verhulst S, Colliver JA, et al. A template for reliable assessment of resident operative performance: assessment intervals, numbers of cases and raters. Surgery 2012;152(4):517–24 [discussion: 524–7].

23. Williams RG, Sanfey H, Chen XP, et al. A controlled study to determine measurement conditions necessary for a reliable and valid operative performance assessment: a controlled prospective observational study. Ann Surg 2012;256(1):177–87.

24. Williams RG, Chen XP, Sanfey H, et al. The measured effect of delay in completing operative performance ratings on clarity and detail of ratings assigned. J Surg Educ 2014;71(6):e132–8.

25. Reznick R, Regehr G, MacRae H, et al. Testing technical skill via an innovative "bench station" examination. Am J Surg 1997;173(3):226–30.

26. Macfie RC, Webel AD, Nesbitt JC, et al. "Boot camp" simulator training in open hilar dissection in early cardiothoracic surgical residency. Ann Thorac Surg 2014;97(1):161–6.

27. Sternbach JM, Wang K, El Khoury R, et al. Measuring error identification and recovery skills in surgical residents. Ann Thorac Surg 2017;103(2):663–9.

28. Jensen K, Hansen HJ, Petersen RH, et al. Evaluating competency in video-assisted thoracoscopic surgery (VATS) lobectomy performance using a novel assessment tool and virtual reality simulation. Surg Endosc 2018. [Epub ahead of print].

29. Jensen K, Petersen RH, Hansen HJ, et al. A novel assessment tool for evaluating competence in video-assisted thoracoscopic surgery lobectomy. Surg Endosc 2018;32(10):4173–82.

30. Enter DH, Lee R, Fann JI, et al. "Top Gun" competition: motivation and practice narrows the technical skill gap among new cardiothoracic surgery residents. Ann Thorac Surg 2015;99(3):870–5 [discussion: 875–6].

31. Lee R, Enter D, Lou X, et al. The Joint Council on Thoracic Surgery Education coronary artery assessment tool has high interrater reliability. Ann Thorac Surg 2013;95(6):2064–9 [discussion: 2069–70].

32. Hicks GL Jr, Gangemi J, Angona RE Jr, et al. Cardiopulmonary bypass simulation at the Boot Camp. J Thorac Cardiovasc Surg 2011;141(1):284–92.

33. Sanfey H, Ketchum J, Bartlett J, et al. Verification of proficiency in basic skills for postgraduate year 1 residents. Surgery 2010;148(4):759–66 [discussion: 766–7].

34. DaRosa DA, Zwischenberger JB, Meyerson SL, et al. A theory-based model for teaching and assessing residents in the operating room. J Surg Educ 2013;70(1):24–30.

35. Meyerson SL, Teitelbaum EN, George BC, et al. Defining the autonomy gap: when expectations do not meet reality in the operating room. J Surg Educ 2014;71(6):e64–72.

36. George BC, Teitelbaum EN, Meyerson SL, et al. Reliability, validity, and feasibility of the Zwisch scale for the assessment of intraoperative performance. J Surg Educ 2014;71(6):e90–6.

37. Ten Cate O. Nuts and bolts of entrustable professional activities. J Grad Med Educ 2013;5(1):157–8.

38. Nousiainen MT, Mironova P, Hynes M, et al. Eight-year outcomes of a competency-based residency training program in orthopedic surgery. Med Teach 2018. [Epub ahead of print].

How to Give Effective Formative Feedback in Thoracic Surgery Education

Ara A. Vaporciyan, MD, MHPE

KEYWORDS

• Education • Feedback • Formative • Surgery • Thoracic

KEY POINTS

- Formative feedback informs a learner of the gap between where they are and where they need to be.
- Using models describing how feedback works in K-12 learning, we can predict how we should best apply it in thoracic surgical education.
- Good feedback answers 3 questions: where is the learner headed (goal), how close is the learner (gap), and how can the learner get there faster (efficiency).
- Feedback can target the task, the processes underlying how tasks work or are related, and the trainee's ability to self-regulate his or her own learning.
- A major difference between feedback in early learners and cardiothoracic fellows is how a cardiothoracic learner's close association of performing surgery and self-image can affect feedback's effectiveness.

There is a clear distinction between formative feedback and summative feedback or evaluation. In the simplest definition, formative feedback is *"for"* education, whereas summative feedback is *"of"* education. Formative feedback provides information. Summative feedback, on the other hand, provides a judgment. More specifically, formative feedback helps a learner see what he or she just accomplished along with the consequences of those actions. It presents that information in association with an agreed-on standard that the trainee is attempting to achieve. The exposure of the "gap" between current and envisioned performance is the strength of formative feedback.[1] Repeatedly highlighting this disparity allows the learner to narrow the gap and reach the desired performance.

Although this provides a nice clean definition, the reality is that all learners will ascribe a level of "judgment" to all forms of feedback. Informing a trainee that he or she did not space the stitches evenly during a coronary anastomosis will engender disappointment in most. As we will see, this "personalization" of feedback, both positive and negative, can have significant impact in how effective feedback is in moving a learner toward his or her goal.

To fulfill the intent of this article, I begin by examining the literature on formative feedback (from here on, referred to as simply "feedback"). From this, I identify and present a conceptual framework of how feedback works. In education, conceptual frameworks are akin to a theory in the biological sciences. You need a theory to generalize how something will behave. Thus, with a framework in hand, we can explore how effective feedback delivery in cardiothoracic surgery might be accomplished.

SCIENTIFIC EVIDENCE SUPPORTING THE USE OF FEEDBACK

Rigorous scientific evaluation of feedback delivery in cardiothoracic surgery is unfortunately scant. In

Disclosure Statement: The author has nothing to disclose.
Department of Thoracic and Cardiovascular Surgery, UT MD Anderson Cancer Center, 1515 Holcombe Boulevard, Box 1489, Houston, TX 77030, USA
E-mail address: avaporci@mdanderson.org

Thorac Surg Clin 29 (2019) 249–257
https://doi.org/10.1016/j.thorsurg.2019.03.003
1547-4127/19/© 2019 Elsevier Inc. All rights reserved.

fact, the research on feedback in graduate medical education (GME) in general is limited. In a recent attempt at reviewing the literature on this very topic, Bing-You and colleagues[2] found that the subject, feedback for learners in medical education, was so far-ranging and contained such multiple varied approaches that is was unsuitable for a systematic review. They instead chose to perform a scoping review. Scoping reviews aim to map the existing literature in terms of the volume, nature, and characteristics of the primary research. They tend to be most useful when the topic has not yet been recently reviewed or is of a complex or heterogeneous nature.[3] Their search spanned from 1980 to 2015. After an initial search and 2 subsequent screenings, they had 650 articles for their scoping review. Most (>85%) were published after 2000. Only 192 (35%) articles addressed medical residents, with only 31 specifying residents or fellows in surgery. Most (52%) of the articles described a new or altered curricular approach or intervention involving feedback, but 85% of these did not specify randomization. Another 19% assessed learners' feedback perceptions using surveys, interviews, and focus groups. Finally, another 15% were simply opinion papers by a group or a single author. Their conclusions were that feedback is an important driver of learner improvements, as evidenced by the large body of literature on the subject. However, at least in medical education, what is known about feedback is not based on strong evidence. This has been validated in other reviews as well.[4]

Of course, this is all simply academic activity. It just proves that we do not study feedback effectively, it does not mean we deliver it ineffectively. Unfortunately there is evidence of our lack of effective feedback from studies of trainee and faculty perceptions on the quality of feedback. A survey of surgical trainees and the faculty at the University of Washington validated that all parties value feedback equally and highly; however, in terms of the timing, amount, specificity of feedback, and the proportion of cases in which they received/provided feedback, the faculty had a much higher impression of their skill than did the trainees.[5] In a similar evaluation at McGill University, investigators found significant large differences between faculty and trainees in relation to the timing and effectiveness of feedback.[6]

In contrast to the volume of work produced on the feedback in GME, the work in other areas is prodigious. In fact, in the scoping review, the authors did note that a few articles support the much larger body of literature in K-12 and post-secondary students delineating behaviorist conceptual frameworks of feedback. Although there have been some recent calls to revisit these frameworks' applicability to medical education, it certainly would be valuable for us to be familiar with them as they are the most rigorously studied framework explaining how feedback works.

A CONCEPTUAL FRAMEWORK OF HOW FEEDBACK WORKS
How Does Feedback Work?

There are a number of frameworks that we could use to guide delivery of effective feedback. Most are very granular, addressing classroom teaching or very early learners. But a few are more generalized in their approach and try to span a wide range of learners. I selected one of the models that appears to apply broadly and has been referenced by educators in GME. Hattie and Temperley[7] used a review of the literature to propose a model or framework of how feedback improves learning. As I mentioned earlier, these frameworks are crucial to our ability to predict how an educational technique will behave in other environments. Like theories in the biologic sciences, their strength is improved by testing their predictive ability in those other environments. However, rigorous scientific investigation of feedback is wanting in medical education. Therefore, their framework, based on decades of work by scores of investigators in other fields, should be a good starting point for GME and specifically cardiothoracic surgery.

Although other models exist that are more granular, the model proposed by Hattie and Temperley[7] is simple and should be more readily translated for cardiothoracic surgical education. In fact, the model (**Fig. 1**) begins with a definition of feedback that closely parallels the definition proposed by Ende[1] whose work specifically addressed feedback in medical education. That is, the goal of feedback is to reduce the discrepancies between a learner's current understanding/performance and a desired goal. A trainee, especially early in training, will recognize that he or she cannot perform a specific procedure or generate a treatment plan for a disease as efficiently or accurately as what he or she believes is the appropriate level of performance.

Once a gap like this is recognized, there are a number of maneuvers that can be performed to help reduce that gap. It should be noted that these maneuvers are not dependent on the provision of feedback; some may occur in its absence but certainly all are possible after the provision of feedback. The more effective maneuvers, and the ones we hope to encourage through feedback, are when students increase their effort or use self-identified strategies to help close the gap. This

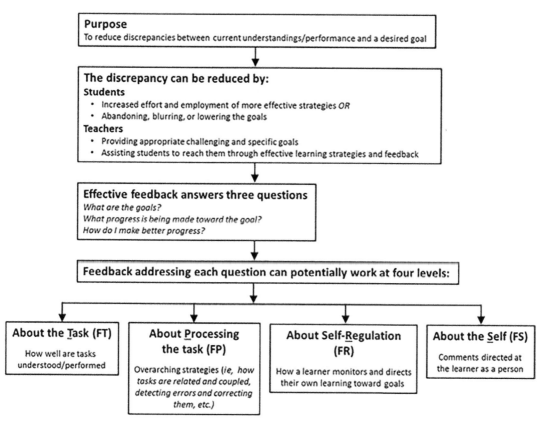

Purpose
To reduce discrepancies between current understandings/performance and a desired goal

The discrepancy can be reduced by:
Students
- Increased effort and employment of more effective strategies OR
- Abandoning, blurring, or lowering the goals

Teachers
- Providing appropriate challenging and specific goals
- Assisting students to reach them through effective learning strategies and feedback

Effective feedback answers three questions
What are the goals?
What progress is being made toward the goal?
How do I make better progress?

Feedback addressing each question can potentially work at four levels:

About the Task (FT)
How well are tasks understood/performed

About Processing the task (FP)
Overarching strategies (*ie, how tasks are related and coupled, detecting errors and correcting them, etc.*)

About Self-Regulation (FR)
How a learner monitors and directs their own learning toward goals

About the Self (FS)
Comments directed at the learner as a person

Fig. 1. A framework of how feedback works to enhance learning. (*Adapted from* Hattie J, Timperley H. The power of feedback. Rev Educ Res 2007;77(1):81–112; with permission.)

behavior is crucial to any expert skill development as identified through research on expertise.[8] This increased effort is consistent with the concept of deliberate practice and it is clearly the ideal we hope to achieve with feedback.

Unfortunately, research also has shown that here are some unproductive strategies that can be initiated by the student to reduce the gap. Kluger and DeNisi[9] highlighted this in their much more detailed proposed framework, Feedback Intervention Theory, and Hattie and Temperley[7] adapted their work into their simplified model. These unproductive strategies range from simply adjusting or blurring the desired goal to overtly abandoning it or rejecting the feedback. For example, consider a trainee presented with a clinical scenario of an intraoperative diagnostic dilemma; say failure to wean from bypass or hypoxia on 1-lung ventilation. The trainee then suggests a set of potential diagnoses but fails to include a rare but possible explanation. In response to the feedback, the trainee should be encouraged to learn more about that diagnosis but may instead choose to rationalize that such a rare disorder is so uncommon that its exclusion will have little impact on most patients' outcome

and thus it really is not necessary to provide competent care. In such a way, the trainee can modify the standard.

Completely abandoning the standard is, of course, a more radical response. In its most egregious form, the trainee abandons the pursuit of cardiothoracic surgery altogether. More commonly, the trainee deems a certain skill unnecessary to his or her overall education and decides not to expend the energy needed to develop that skill. Consider congenital cardiac surgery. Faced with a significant gap in performance in selecting the appropriate treatments, some trainees may simply abandon this goal.

Rejecting the feedback also can occur. This appears more common when the feedback is in direct conflict with the way the learners view themselves. More on this later, but in short, trainees tend to reject or ignore negative feedback that contradicts their self-assessment. Everyone can recall an example of an overconfident trainee. When faced with negative feedback, these individuals are more likely to reject that feedback. Rejection is even easier when prior feedback has included generalized nonconstructive praise (eg, "You did a good job").

Hattie and Temperley[7] also highlight ways that teachers can influence the effectiveness of feedback. Providing specific goals that push trainees just beyond their comfort zone is the most direct strategy. Key to this strategy is the specificity of the goals.[10] The most common way this guideline is unfulfilled is in the feedback provided with end-of-rotation evaluations. Telling a trainee he or she is "still having trouble with esophageal cancer management" will have little impact on learning. On the other hand, being specific about where the difficulty exists, such as in the diagnosis, staging, or selection of treatments, is much more effective. If problems exist in multiple domains, then specifying which one the trainee should focus on first is better than describing the much loftier goal of correcting the entire gap.

In addition, teachers can provide learning strategies to enhance the trainees' ability to close the gap. They can enhance the trainees' commitment toward the goals and they can help trainees develop the skills to self-regulate and detect errors on their own. The remainder of Hattie and Timperley's model[7] is focused on just how feedback can be delivered to increase the productive maneuvers.

How Is Feedback Delivered?

All forms of feedback include, to some degree, answers to 3 questions, as shown in **Fig. 2**. The first question defines the goals. All goals have 2 dimensions: challenge and commitment. The challenge is the characteristic element of a goal. It includes the details of the understanding/performance desired in the trainee. The more specific such details are, the less "wiggle" room is available. Recall how some trainees may adjust or blur the goal in response to the feedback. The commitment dimension is the "why" of a goal. The most common and effective techniques, especially in the medical professions, is role modeling. Of course, in medicine there are also clear incentives and rewards for reaching a goal and punishments for failing to reach them. Both of these also provide a commitment.

The second question is what most of us think of when we envision feedback. Where is the trainee in relation to the goal? Here is where we will deliver the constructive task-focused information to illuminate the size of the gap between a trainee's current performance and the goal we outlined in the first question. Without information regarding the first question, the data provided in response to this question will be difficult to benchmark.

The final question is how to help the trainee translate the feedback into efficient progress toward the goal. Usually the response here is to simply "do more." Of course the more granular the goal and specific the feedback on the progress, the easier it is to decide where more should be done. As shown in the next section, feedback can and should be specifically focused here to create self-regulating learners who can identify their own deficiencies and initiate their own learning strategies to address them.

As you can see, all 3 of these questions are dependent on each other. Without clear goals, any feedback on progress has no reference criterion. Without guidance on what they might do to address the gap, the efficiency with which it is closed is reduced. So if the intent of feedback is to improve progress toward a goal, then addressing all 3 questions is paramount.

Where Is Feedback Focused?

The model by Hattie and Timperley[7] claims 4 major levels of focus for feedback. as shown in **Fig. 2**. The most common, and what most of us think of when we envision feedback, is feedback about the task (FT). Often called "corrective," FT points out the discrepancy between the performance of a task and a standard at which it should be performed. This is the most basic form of feedback. Its power is enhanced when it identifies faulty interpretation of data rather than simply a lack of knowledge. For example, a trainee reviews a computed tomography scan of a mediastinal mass and fails to order the proper laboratory tests in his or her evaluation. Rather than simply telling the trainee that he or she failed to order the correct laboratory tests, an improved form of FT would be to explain the faulty interpretation of the differential of a mediastinal mass. FT also can be enhanced by coupling it with the next 2 levels: feedback on processing tasks (FP) and feedback directed at self-regulation (FR). If all feedback focuses only on tasks, the trainee may focus on the minutia and avoid the larger picture. Trainees may move toward a more "trial-and-error" approach simply to fulfill the focused task performance and fail to integrate that task with others toward the overarching goal.

Unfortunately, some approaches diminish the power of FT. Complex FT is less effective than simple FT. Rather than explaining the entire literature on the treatment options for mitral valve disease when a trainee fails to select the correct treatment plan, a more focused simplistic FT on the specifics of the plan the trainee provided would be more effective. Similarly, FT mixed with feedback that engages a trainee's self-image (FS) dilutes the power of FT, and for that

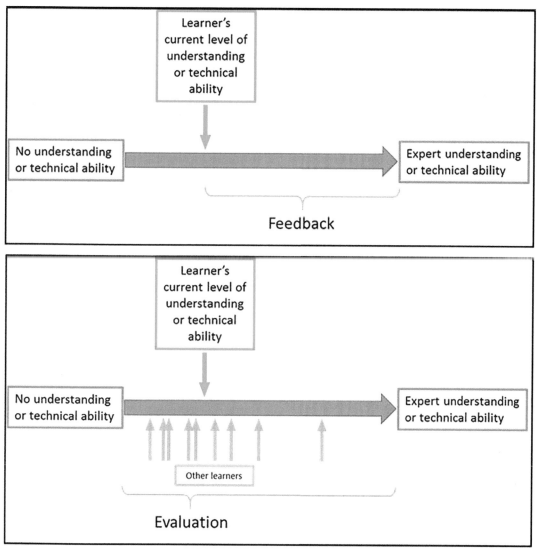

Fig. 2. The difference between providing feedback (*top*) and providing an evaluation (*bottom*). Feedback focuses on the gap between where a learner is and where they are headed. It also focuses on how to bridge or narrow that gap. An evaluation, on the other hand, shows a learner where he or she is along the entire continuum of learning about a topic. It can also provide input on how they compare to other learners. It provides a much broader summative view.

matter, all forms of feedback. In fact, there is even considerable evidence that grades, when combined with feedback, tend to diminish learning.

FP is the next level and focuses on how various tasks are linked toward a goal. Although one task may be accurate staging of lung cancer, understanding how staging influences subsequent tasks like treatment planning is an example of FP. It helps trainees understand that they are doing this to allow/prevent/enable this subsequent goal. Providing FP along with FT enhances the power of both forms of feedback.

The next level, actually the highest level, is FR. This addresses how a trainee monitors, directs, and regulates actions toward a goal. This skill is central to the core competency of practice-based learning and improvement, the idea that we will train surgeons who continually seek to improve themselves. When you provide FR, be aware that there are 6 major factors that affect how trainees self-regulate. Briefly they include the ability to self-assess, the willingness to seek out and deal with feedback, the trainees' confidence in their ability, personal attributions regarding success or failure, the impact of effort versus ability, and finally the type of help they seek. When providing FP, these are the areas in which you should focus it.

Self-assessment includes both the ability to self-assess (find the errors) and self-manage (fix or minimize errors). Less effective learners will rely heavily on external feedback. Willingness to seek out or deal with feedback is based on the trainee weighing the benefit of the feedback against a variety of "costs." These include the effort needed to receive the feedback, how they will be perceived because they asked for feedback, and the potential of misinterpreting the feedback.[11] If these trainees feel any of these "costs" are too high, they will refrain from gathering feedback.

Their confidence level also influences how trainees interpret and weigh feedback. There is a relationship between the effectiveness of feedback versus providing additional knowledge that is influenced by the level of confidence a trainee might have. In general, if trainees think they understand a concept like weaning a patient from bypass, when they make an error they are very eager to correct that error and are thus receptive to feedback. On the other hand, if they decannulate properly, any feedback they receive is likely to be ignored. Conversely, if they have low confidence in their ability and perform poorly, feedback will be less motivational. Even if they perform well, they will have some response but little motivation to change. Instead, in these latter 2 groups, more instruction is the better approach. Note that high confidence here is different from the overconfidence described earlier.

The trainees' attributions toward success and failure also can influence how they respond to feedback. If both are not clearly tied to the goals, some trainees may over interpret both failures and successes. Feedback on effort appears to be more valuable when first learning a skill. Once the skill is more developed, feedback on ability may be more beneficial. Finally, there are 2 levels of help a trainee can seek: instrumental and executive. The former is looking for hints, whereas the latter is looking for answers to avoid time and work. Clearly, the goal is to provide FR to enhance the former rather than the latter.

The last focus of feedback is directed toward the self as a person (FS). Hattie and Timperley[7] included it in their model not because it is effective, but rather because it is detrimental and used, unfortunately, frequently. It includes the oft-used phrases like "good job," or "well done." It is also sometimes negative. Unfortunately, volumes of research have shown that it is rarely converted into more engagement, commitment, self-efficacy, or understanding about the task.[12] In fact, some investigators have shown that simply avoiding praise has a greater

impact on learning.[9] However, there is a very important distinction. Praise directed away from the task and toward the learner is ineffective. Praise specifically about the task and its proper performance is another form of FT, FP, and FS and is clearly effective. This is not to say that students do not appreciate praise. However, as a method to improve learning, it has little benefit.

APPLYING THE MODEL TO CARDIOTHORACIC SURGERY TRAINING

I remind the readers that the model described previously was not developed in GME. As such, it has not been tested and validated in our learners. Still, it is backed by a wealth of controlled experimental data in comparison with the less rigorous data supporting some of the nonbehaviorist models offered by medical educators. Still, some consistent discrepancies have been observed and these should be discussed and potentially included in any guidelines.

Impact of Self-Image on Acceptance of Feedback

The link between performance and one's self-image appears to be closer among medical learners than seen in nonmedical learners.[13] Strong emotional reactions can occur among physicians when feedback contradicts their own self-assessment. Unlike K-12 learners, medical learners, and especially those in GME, have invested significant effort in getting where they are. A sophomore in high school is unlikely to have his self-image shaken by negative feedback in algebra class. However, a cardiothoracic surgical trainee's self-image is heavily tied to his or her role as a surgeon. Thus, feedback that undermines that self-image can be very difficult to accept.[14] In fact, some of the very strengths of feedback may actually undermine elements related to self-determination, a sense of competence, autonomy, and connectedness to others. For example, repeated feedback may diminish a trainees' intrinsic motivation by eroding their feeling of competence. This may be a greater factor in earlier learners in residencies rather than fellowships and may explain the higher rates of attrition seen in residencies.[15] Unfortunately, evidence-based research is limited in this area and is nonexistent in fellowship-based training paradigms like cardiothoracic surgery.[16,17]

Value of Rapport with and Credibility of the Instructor

The importance of the relationship between the teacher and the trainee and the conversational nature of feedback delivery,[13,18] along with how a learner perceives the credibility of the teacher, affects the willingness of the trainee to accept feedback.[19] Our learners have amassed a significant volume of knowledge and feel closer to their teachers than say interns do to their general surgery faculty (or that sophomore to the algebra teacher). When one considers the impact on self-image discussed previously, a cardiothoracic surgical trainee may be quite selective in who he or she will be willing to accept feedback from. If the credibility or relationship is deemed weak, the trainee is unlikely to accept negative feedback. Going back to the model presented earlier, non-credible sources are much more likely to lead to unproductive responses to feedback, specifically rejection.

Timing

A wealth of literature in both the behaviorist and GME communities has shown that delivery of feedback is most effective when it is given in close proximity to the event. That being said, there are some practical considerations that must be taken into account; primarily is the safety of the patient and other health care workers. However, another important consideration is the impact on self-image. Both negative and even positive feedback, when delivered publicly in front of peers, can magnify any threats to a learner's self-image. The goal is to illuminate the gap in the learner's progress, not crush his or her self-image and erase the motivation to learn.

HOW TO DELIVER FEEDBACK

So where does that leave us? How do we apply this evidence-based model in our day-to-day practice of training fellows and residents? Unfortunately, the medical literature is awash with various rubrics to help medical educators deliver feedback. These include, but are not limited to, REFLECT[20] (Reflection Evaluation for Learners' Enhanced Competencies Tool), FAIRness[21] (feedback, activity, relevance, and individualization), RIME[22] (reporter-interpreter-manager-educator), and PEARLS[23] (partnership, empathy, apology, respect, legitimation, support). Most of these leverage the criticisms leveraged against the behaviorist approaches we discussed earlier. They highlight the discrepancies we pointed out in the preceding section. However, the weight of evidence and the generalizability of these methods is very limited. Some are based entirely on focus groups by faculty with minimal data demonstrating an impact on learning. Despite these limitations, there are clearly some guidelines based on this

work that make intuitive sense and should be considered. Some even can link back to the behaviorist models we initially discussed. These guidelines are integral to many of the models listed previously and many authors have provided guidelines such as these.[1,23,24] A condensed list appears in **Table 1**.

Although these guidelines are helpful, the evidence-based data we have from the behaviorist models should still provide the foundation for most of the day-to-day feedback we deliver. Cardiothoracic surgical trainees are most commonly a heavily motivated group. Visualizing where they are in their progress toward a mutually accepted goal is often eagerly desired. Doing that effectively and efficiently is to everyone's benefit. **Fig. 3** simplifies what we learned from a behaviorist's model

Table 1 Guidelines	
Guidelines	**Description**
Always base feedback on personal observations	The less data driven the feedback, the less credible the source.
Use neutral statements tied to you as an observer	"I saw you do…" and "I noticed that…" rather than "You can't…" or "You didn't…" The focus is on your observations, not on the trainee as a person.
Tie it to a goal	Focus on highlighting their progress toward a goal.
Ask for their thoughts before and after	This is linked to feedback about self-reflection and can help develop their self-assessment and management skills.
Consider the timing and locations of delivery	Minimize the impact on their self-image by choosing carefully where the feedback is delivered.
Create a consistent culture of feedback delivery	If it happens consistently and uniformly, the stigma associated with its episodic delivery will be reduced.

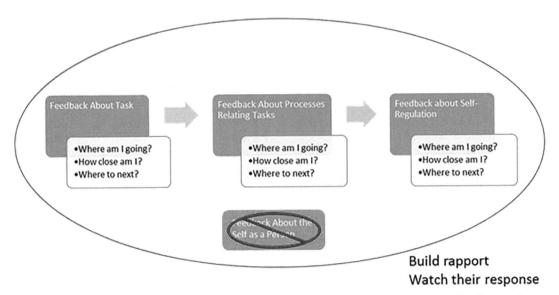

Fig. 3. A model of effective formative feedback delivery in thoracic surgical education. Target feedback at 3 separate domains: a task, processes about tasks or how tasks are related, and finally how the learner self-regulates the ability to obtain and use feedback as well as learn. Avoid feedback targeting the learner as an individual. In each domain, always provide information on the goal, the gap between their current progress and the goal, and ways they can close the gap efficiently. Remember to build rapport and to watch their response. Be cognizant of the tendency of GME learners to disregard feedback that contradicts their self-image with their self-image.

of feedback delivery and can serve as a set of guidelines for GME educators. Remember the 3 domains in which feedback should be targeted: the immediate task being performed, the relationship and processes involved in the performance of task(s), and the ability to self-regulate one's own learning. When targeting these domains, remember to address the 3 questions that make feedback effective: where am I going, how close am I, and where to next? Remember that although feedback about the task is often the easiest and most common domain we target, the ability for feedback to deeply affect learning is magnified when this feedback is accompanied by feedback in the other 2 domains. Always omit feedback targeting the learner as an individual. Minimize anything that leads them to reflect the feedback toward their self-image. This will simply increase the unproductive responses to feedback. Finally, provide the feedback in an environment in which you build rapport and consistent environment in which feedback is the norm. Carefully observe their response, being mindful of the unproductive responses to feedback that trainees can implement.

SUMMARY

Feedback is a powerful tool to assist learning. In our existing approach to GME, feedback is probably one of the most effective tools we have,

especially for teaching the complex concepts surrounding clinical decision-making we must pass on. Anytime feedback is not provided, or even provided poorly, we have wasted an opportunity. Evidence-based research on how feedback works, and also does not work, can and should be used to guide its effective delivery in GME. Models derived from that research, mostly derived from younger learners, are an excellent resource to guide how to deliver effective feedback. Still we should recognize that there may be some differences based on the types of learners we are working with.

I hope this work has also made it clear that the proper delivery of feedback is a skill, and like most skills is not something we are all born with. Most of us infrequently experienced properly delivered feedback during our training or, almost certainly, were exposed to flawed attempts at feedback delivery. Unfortunately, when new graduates suddenly take on the role of teachers, their skill in feedback delivery is mostly based on what they were exposed to. This perpetuates the existence of poor feedback delivery in future teacher-learner interaction. To become more effective teachers, we must all understand what good feedback includes and how best to deliver it.

Finally, there is a wide gap in our understanding of how feedback works in higher levels of GME. Further research is needed to test the applicability of models derived from early K-12 learners. An even wider gulf exists when we think of feedback delivery during continuing medical education. I hope that future generations of cardiothoracic surgeons will recognize that research in this area is a fruitful area of investigation and begin to slowly address these gaps.

REFERENCES

1. Ende J. Feedback in clinical medical education. JAMA 1983;250:777–81.

2. Bing-You R, Hayes V, Varaklis K, et al. Feedback for learners in medical education: what is known? A scoping review. Acad Med 2017;92(9):1346–54.

3. Pham MT, Rajic A, Greig JD, et al. A scoping review of scoping reviews: advancing the approach and enhancing the consistency. Res Synth Methods 2014,5.371–85.

4. van de Ridder JMM, McGaghie WC, Stokking KM, et al. Variables that affect the process and outcome of feedback, relevant for medical training: a meta-review. Med Educ 2015;49:658–73.

5. Jenson AR, Wright AS, Kim S, et al. Educational feedback in the operating room: a gap between resident and faculty perceptions. Am J Surg 2012;204: 248–55.

6. Liberman AS, Liberman M, Steinert Y, et al. Surgery residents and attending surgeons have different perceptions of feedback. Med Teach 2005;27(5):470–2.

7. Hattie J, Timperley H. The power of feedback. Rev Educ Res 2007;77(1):81–112.

8. Ericsson KA. Deliberate practice and the acquisition and maintenance of expert performance in medicine and related domains. Acad Med 2004;79(10): S70–81.

9. Kluger AN, DeNisi A. The effect of feedback interventions on performance: a historical review, a meta-analysis, and a preliminary feedback intervention theory. Psychol Bull 1996;119(2):254–84.

10. Locke EA, Latham GP. Goal setting: a motivational technique that works. Englewood Cliffs (NJ): Prentice Hall; 1984.

11. De Luque MF, Sommer SM. The impact of culture on feed-back-seeking behavior: an integrated model and propositions. Acad Manage Rev 2000;25(4): 829–49.

12. Wilkinson SS. The relationship of teacher praise and student achievement: a meta-analysis of selected research. Dissertation Abstracts International 1981; 461(9-A):3998.

13. Sargeant J, Lockyer J, Mann K, et al. Facilitated reflective performance feedback: developing and evidence-and theory-based model that builds relationship, explores reactions and content, and coaches for performance change (R2C2). Acad Med 2015;90:1698–706.

14. Cate OTJ. Why receiving feedback collides with self determination. Adv Health Sci Educ Theory Pract 2013;18:845–9.

15. Dodson TF, Webb AL. Why do residents leave general surgery? The hidden problem in today's programs. Curr Surg 2005;62:128–31.

16. Sargeant J, Mann K, Sinclair D, et al. Tensions in informed self-assessment: how the desire for feedback and reticence to collect and use it can conflict. Acad Med 2011;86:1120–7.

17. Sargeant J, Mann K, Sinclair D, et al. Understanding the influence of emotions and reflection upon multisource feedback acceptance and use. Adv Health Sci Educ Theory Pract 2008;13:275–88.

18. Johnson CE, Keating JL, Boud DJ, et al. Identifying educator behaviors for high quality verbal feedback in health professions education: literature review and expert refinement. Med Educ 2016;16(96):1–11.

19. Bing-You RG, Paterson J, Levin MA. Feedback falling on deaf ears: residents' receptivity to feedback tempered by sender credibility. Med Teach 1997; 19(1):40–3.

20. Wald HS, Reis SP, Monroe AD, et al. "The loss of my elderly patient:" interactive reflective writing to support medical students' rites of passage. Med Teach 2010;32:e178–84.

21. Chan P. FAIRness and clinical teaching. Med Teach 2013;35:779–81.

22. DeWitt D, Carline J, Paauw D, et al. Pilot study of a "RIME"-based tool for giving feedback in a multispecialty longitudinal clerkship. Med Educ 2008; 42:1205–9.

23. Milan FB, Parish SJ, Reichgott MJ. A model for educational feedback based on clinical communication skills strategies: beyond the "feedback sandwich". Teach Learn Med 2006;18:42–7.

24. Ramani S, Krackov SK. Twelve tips for giving feedback effectively in the clinical environment. Med Teach 2012;34:787–91.

Unconscious Bias
Addressing the Hidden Impact on Surgical Education

Leah M. Backhus, MD, MPH[a],*, Natalie S. Lui, MD, MAS[a],
David T. Cooke, MD[b], Errol L. Bush, MD[c],
Zachary Enumah, MD[c], Robert Higgins, MD, MSHA[c]

KEYWORDS

• Unconscious bias • Implicit bias • Hidden brain • Disparities • Bias training

KEY POINTS

- Unconscious biases serve as mental shortcuts to allow us to make efficient decisions, which is valuable to the cardiothoracic surgeon.
- Unconscious bias is ubiquitous and affects all aspects of cardiothoracic surgery education from medical student applicants, to resident trainees, and the faculty who teach them.
- Unconscious bias has several unintended negative consequences that influence trainee selection, how we teach trainees, and what we teach them in patient interactions.
- The Implicit Association Test is one tool that can help identify unconscious biases that has been widely studied.
- Individuals must acknowledge the presence of unconscious biases and their effects, whereas institutions must provide a framework for culture change and capitalize on many of the training resources available to create a diverse academic environment.

INTRODUCTION

Unconscious (or implicit) biases are learned stereotypes that are automatic, unintentional, deeply engrained, universal, and able to influence behavior.[1] We are all subject to unconscious bias (UB). It is ubiquitous with deep evolutionary roots reinforced by lived experiences and social determinants. These attitudes lie outside of our awareness and extend beyond race and ethnicity. Some characteristics often subject to UB include sexual orientation groups, gender, weight, age, social class, and even height. Why then have we

evolved to rely on and reinforce biases for important decisions rather than sound empirical data? The reality is that our biases help expedite decision making and often even work to our advantage. By definition, UB lives within our unconscious or the "hidden brain." The hidden brain has evolved to be highly efficient and, in many instances, sacrifices sophistication for the sake of speed. As an example, by 3 months of age, human infants demonstrate a strong bias toward human faces.[2] From an evolutionary standpoint, one can appreciate the potential protective benefits of such a bias. The precise reasons for this bias in

Disclosure Statement: The authors have nothing to disclose.
[a] Stanford University, 300 Pasteur Drive, Falk Research Building, Stanford, CA 94304, USA; [b] UC Davis Health, 2335 Stockton Blvd, Suite 6121, North Addition Office Building, Sacramento, CA 95817, USA; [c] Johns Hopkins University School of Medicine, Johns Hopkins University, 720 Rutland Avenue, Ross 759, Baltimore, MD 21205, USA
* Corresponding author. Department of Cardiothoracic Surgery, Stanford University, 300 Pasteur Drive, Falk Research Building, Stanford, CA 94304.
E-mail address: lbackhus@stanford.edu

infants remain unclear. One hypothesis is that we as humans have adapted to favor "things" that are "like" us. Problems arise, however, when our UB influence our decisions in the absence of affirming data rendering them at best inaccurate and at worst, harmful.

The discipline of medicine is no exception to the influence of UB. Several studies have documented the effects of provider biases on patient care and outcomes. "[Assumptions] can narrow the options a physician gives the… patients and this limits a patient's opportunity to make a well-informed decision," (Laura Castillo-Page, PhD, Association of American Medical Colleges [AAMC] senior director for diversity policy and programs). But the implications of UB in medicine extend beyond that of the individual patient. They include issues regarding graduate and undergraduate medical education and the pipeline of trainees entering into the academic medical faculty. This article provides a framework for exploring the implications for UB in surgical education and highlight best practices toward minimizing its impact.

A great deal of medical education comes in the form of pattern recognition. A patient who is a certain age and presents with a certain symptom set triggers a well-defined differential diagnosis and anticipated work-up and treatment. Stereotypes of diseases are one of the cornerstones of medical education and allow us to acquire and synthesize a large volume of information and expeditiously arrive at a diagnosis and treatment plan. In the realm of cardiothoracic surgery, we are often working under time pressure that requires all of the previously mentioned processes to occur in a compressed timeframe with immediate consequences. The intensity of a cardiothoracic operation demands efficiency in decision making, which is often based on prior experience and anticipation. These are extremely beneficial to the cardiothoracic surgeon.

Furthermore, the surgeon in training must progress through defined stages of technical skill acquisition. In moving from novice to master, the surgeon relies on their ability to hard-wire technical steps and decision making into their work. Successfully anticipating challenges during the conduct of an operation requires the surgeon to use stereotyped pattern recognition while safely addressing technical challenges and the use of muscle memory. Both of these allow the expert surgeon to be safe and efficient. Stereotypes are ingrained as mental shortcuts that are valuable to our work and the way we teach it to our trainees.

The dilemma is, that in teaching medicine and surgery, we instill thinking processes and manual tasks with repetition such that they become rote.

We want to capitalize on the ability of the brain to automate complex functions so that we are quicker and more efficient at doing our work. We teach pattern recognition as a short cut and repetition as a means of quality control. Yet, these same behaviors are rooted in making rapid assumptions and when those assumptions become embedded in our subconscious, they are indeed biases by definition. Thus, not all UB are harmful. Our biases cross the line and become counterproductive when (1) they perpetuate or validate existing disparities in our world and more acutely in cardiothoracic surgery, (2) they affect how we teach, or (3) they affect what we teach. How then to harness the benefits of unconscious thinking, yet consciously reflect on our behavior and root out the negative UB that can undermine our best efforts? First, we must identify the problem. What are the UBs that are counterproductive to our mission?

DEFINING THE PROBLEM: IMPACT OF UNCONSCIOUS BIAS ON SURGICAL EDUCATION
The Surgical Education Pipeline

Addressing the role that UB plays at every level is paramount in recruiting and training the next generation of surgical leaders. Diversity of appearance breeds diversity in experience. Yet, the current medical landscape still has improvements to make along the pipeline to creating a more diverse surgical workforce. Women and minorities have long been underrepresented in medicine, especially in cardiothoracic surgery. Currently, women comprise about 48% of medical school students, 41% of general surgery residents, and 20% of cardiothoracic surgery residents.[3] In 2014 to 2015, African Americans represented 12.4% of the United States population, 5.7% of medical students, and 6.2% of general surgery residents.[4] In the same years, Hispanics represented 17.4% of the United States population, 4.5% of medical students, and 8.5% of general surgery residents.[4] It is important that we study how UB affects graduate and undergraduate medical education and for many, the point of entry into the educational pipeline is medical school admissions.

Implications for Undergraduate and Medical Education

Given the shift in many cardiothoracic training programs toward the integrated 6-year training format, undergraduate education has garnered increasing importance in feeding the cardiothoracic surgery workforce. Studies have demonstrated that UB plays a significant role in recruiting and practice across disciplines and fields including criminal justice, education, and health care but precise measurement is challenging.[5–7] One measure of UB that has been studied extensively is the Implicit Association Test (IAT) developed by social psychologists. The IAT is a computer-based tool that requires subjects to quickly categorize two target concepts with an attribute (eg, the concepts "male" and "female" with the attribute "logical"), such that easier pairings generate quicker response times and are interpreted as more strongly associated in memory thus more congruent with biases.[8] Strong gender and race preferences are often revealed by those who take the test. In a study conducted at the Ohio State University, 140 members of the medical school admissions committee took the black–white IAT. Researchers found that all groups (men, women, students, and faculty) displayed significant levels of implicit white preference, with males and faculty demonstrating the largest bias measures. The benefit of the test was that 67% of survey respondents believed that knowing their IAT results might be helpful in reducing bias in medical school admissions.[9] The IAT is not universally accepted as the gold standard for assessing UB with some pointing out low reproducibility and difficulty in interpretation. Nonetheless it remains the most validated instrument available and still likely has utility in identifying and targeting biases.

The effects of UB on undergraduate medical education also has the potential to influence student specialty choice. van Ryn and coworkers[10] explored this issue among medical students at the Mayo Clinic College of Medicine and found that when medical students are exposed to negative comments from attending physicians, their own negative implicit attitudes can worsen. Negative biases from faculty can also influence the way students are taught to treat and interact with patients. A study of first-year medical students at Johns Hopkins noted results from an IAT measuring weight bias, and demonstrated that 70% of students held a "thin" preference. Perhaps more concerning, however, were the biases held by students who believed that obesity was the result of ignorance (74%) and laziness (28%).[11] The influence of UB on medical care has also been well documented. The Institute of Medicine report, Unequal Treatment published in 2002, detailed significant variation in the rates of medical procedures by race, even when insurance status, income, age, and severity of conditions are comparable.[12] It includes disparities in diagnosis and treatment of conditions ranging from acute coronary syndromes, rates of limb amputation among patients with diabetes, addressing postoperative or acute pain, and delivery of cancer care services. The underpinnings of these disparities may lie in UBs that are transferred to impressionable trainees.

Implications for Graduate Medical Education

Almost assuredly the same biases affecting medical school admissions are mirrored at the level of resident selection, but there may be other nuanced differences for the cardiothoracic surgical resident. A study of medical student applicants seeking cardiothoracic surgery residency positions demonstrated that despite being academically successful, many students experience significant negativity regarding their applications depending on whether they are applying to both general surgery and cardiothoracic surgery versus integrated thoracic residency programs alone. This bias can originate from either the general surgery or thoracic surgery faculty and is not lost on the applicant.[13] Another potential bias is in the form of geographic preference. Although some applicants may feel more "welcome" at their home institution, the reverse can also be felt. One study quantified the effect of "homefield advantage" in that one-quarter of categorical general surgery slots were filled with "home program" graduates. Such a preference is intuitive, but does nothing to advance a diverse experiential educational environment critical for learning.[14]

Many studies have focused on better understanding the presence and implications for UB in surgical residency with regards to gender (**Box 1**).[15,16] In 1996, Dresler and colleagues[17] published their results of a survey mailed to all women and a cohort of men certified by the American Board of Thoracic Surgery. Women reported significantly more discrimination during their cardiothoracic residency training. The sources of discrimination were female and male attendings, female and male resident colleagues, nurses, staff, and patients or families. Women were also significantly more likely to believe that gender

---

Box 1
Examples of biased comments

- "She's too nice to be a cardiac surgeon."
- "She's technically very good. She operates like a man!"
- "Women should consider other surgical subspecialties instead of cardiothoracic surgery, since the lifestyle is better."
- "This needle is way too small – it's for girls!"

bias had hindered their career. More recently, Bruce and colleagues[18] surveyed members of the Association of Women Surgeons. Of 334 female medical students, residents, and practicing physicians, 87% experienced gender-based discrimination in medical school, 88% in residency, and 91% in practice. Myers and colleagues[19] interviewed general surgery residents in an academic center. They found that female residents were less likely to self-identify as a "surgeon" (11% vs 38%; *P*<.001) and believed their professional role was disregarded more often by patients and physicians.

Surveys have also addressed race-based discrimination and inequities in surgical training. Wong and colleagues[20] reviewed survey results from general surgery residents taking the 2008 American Board of Surgery In-Training Examination. African American and Asian residents were less likely to believe that they fit in at their programs compared with white residents (73.9% vs 83.3% vs 86.2%). African American residents were less likely to believe they could count on their peers for help (85.2% vs 77.2%). Although these results may not seem to influence resident training at first glance, they are integral to supporting physician well-being and add to other microaggressions experienced disproportionately by these groups. Importantly, they contribute to physician burnout and attrition at every level.

Evaluating evaluations

Gender bias has also been studied in reviewing resident evaluations. Dayal and colleagues[21] studied resident milestone evaluations by faculty at several emergency medicine residency programs. They found that female and male residents had similar milestone levels initially, but male residents had a 12.7% higher rate of milestone attainment through the 3-year program. By the last year of training, male residents were rated higher than female residents for all 23 subcompetencies. There was no difference in evaluations between female and male faculty.

Mueller and colleagues[22] expanded on the previous study by reviewing the qualitative assessments of residents. They found that male residents with poor evaluations received consistent feedback from different faculty, whereas female residents with poor evaluations received inconsistent feedback. In addition, this inconsistent feedback often involved issues of autonomy and assertiveness. In contrast to these qualitative assessments, bias was not apparent in quantitative assessments of the same residents underscoring the need for more objectivity and standardization in resident evaluations.[15,23]

Operative autonomy

Teaching the technical conduct of an operation is a complex interplay between resident and attending surgeon and is difficult to objectively measure. One measure that has been studied is that of operative autonomy and research examining gender bias in this area has been mixed. Meyerson and colleagues[24] studied thoracic surgery residents and faculty who evaluated intraoperative autonomy using the four-point Zwisch scale. Faculty reported that female residents had less autonomy than male residents (30% vs 37%) and female residents reported lower autonomy compared with male residents (19% vs 33% with meaningful autonomy). In contrast, Thompson-Burdine and colleagues[25] examined faculty entrustment and resident entrustability scores across several surgical specialties using the OpTrust scoring system. They found that resident sex was not associated with faculty entrustment in the operating room. Among recent female graduates of cardiothoracic training programs, women were equally satisfied with their career choice, had similar numbers of interviews and job offers, and felt equally prepared for their boards. However, they felt less prepared technically and less ready for independent practice, highlighting a deficit in our training techniques or a failure to instill confidence where it is appropriate. Either explanation represents room for improvement.[26]

Implications for Surgical Faculty

One of the most critical elements to diversify the workforce is to have supportive faculty and leadership, who have a diversity of ideas and backgrounds. Thus, lack of diversity in cardiothoracic surgery at the faculty and administrative levels has untoward effects on graduate medical education. There are many reasons contributing to disparities among cardiothoracic academic faculty spanning the continuum of recruitment, promotion, and tenure. Although much attention has been given toward early stage medical trainees, comparatively less effort and has been devoted to the ranks of the surgical faculty.

Faculty recruitment and retention

There are several negative consequences for lack of cultural diversity among faculty affecting the institution, its individuals, and the overall clinical and educational mission. The problem is fueled by high attrition rates with loss of great talent when an underrepresented minority (URM) is not considered for promotion in a timely manner or leaves the institution, academia, or medicine. Retention is one of the first things that must be addressed before change is contemplated. Rodriguez and colleagues[27] identified issues contributing to URM faculty attrition and highlighted lack of mentorship access, peer networks, professional skill development, and understanding of institutional culture as recurring themes. A recent longitudinal analysis of AAMC and Accreditation Council of Graduate Medical Education data since 2005 detailed this lack of diversity in surgical faculty.[28] The authors identified that for African Americans, at all ranks of the academic ladder, including tenure, there was either no change or a decrease in represented proportions. For Hispanic faculty, except for assistant professors where there was significant proportional decrease, all other ranks, including tenure, experienced significant increases in the represented proportions of members. These findings suggest that although diversification initiatives may be effective in producing positive change in some areas, the effects are not unanimously appreciated, and that particular additional focus may be necessary to include certain URM groups.

Once recruited, faculty are subject to the same UB that affect surgical trainees, but they also experience UB in unique ways with implications for patient care and professional advancement. In one compelling example, Files and colleagues[29] reviewed whether professional titles were used when introducing speakers at internal medicine grand rounds. They found that female introducers were more likely to use professional titles compared with male introducers (96% vs 66%), and male introducers were more likely to use professional titles when introducing male speakers compared with female speakers (72% vs 49%). Furthermore, female faculty may be subject to different evaluation criteria even from their surgical trainees. In a study by Fassiotto and colleagues,[30] female physician faculty received lower evaluations than their male counterparts across all specialties but the negative effects were most pronounced for female physicians being evaluated in specialties with low female representation. Bias may also influence the norms for evaluating surgeon competency such that referring physicians may view surgical outcomes more adversely when performed by female surgeons, reflected by a sharper decrease in subsequent referrals. This has the potential for dire consequences for surgical revenue and overall standing within departments.[31,32] It also has the potential to affect the way a female faculty member may teach within the operating room in terms of resident surgical autonomy if she perceives heightened scrutiny.

STRATEGIES TO ADDRESS THE ISSUES

Ultimately, we would like to catalyze change within our entire specialty toward improving the quality of the surgeons we train and the quality of patient care (**Box 2**). Many psychology experiments that seek to change UB of individuals take an approach akin to treating UB as something like diabetes: a chronic condition that is managed, not a behavior to overcome. Approaching the issue from the standpoint of viewing all UB as "bad," labels all those who harbor UB as "bad people." But physicians are often seen as an egalitarian group, thus acknowledging our own biases and the way in which they may negatively impact the care of patients or teaching of residents is a difficult prospect to grapple with. This concept is called cognitive dissonance and serves as one of the potential barriers to change. By divorcing the concept of bias as indicative of maleficence, only then will individuals and institutions be successful in attempts to overcome them.

Targeted Strategies for Trainees

There are other barriers to overcoming bias that are specific to the training paradigm. First, there is a large power differential between trainees and faculty. Faculty have control over the quality of education, quality of life, subsequent training, and career opportunities of trainees. Residents play an important role in identifying and eliminating UB, yet fear of retaliation means they may not feel empowered to speak out. It is often not until their later years when they have better rapport with attending

---

Box 2
Strategies to address UB in surgical education

- Incorporate IAT into onboarding for faculty and trainees
- Third-party training/workshops for departments and institutions on implicit bias and its impact
- Formal mentoring programs (peer-to-peer and trainee-faculty)
- Blinded promotion practices
- Objective assessments/milestone evaluations
- Transparent, objective compensation plans
- Well-articulated institutional commitment/vision planning
- Structured and objective interview techniques for residency program
- Reporting protocols for perceived bias or discriminatory behavior

physicians that they feel comfortable reporting bias. Many times, the UB may not be obvious such that it is unclear whether bias has contributed at all. Choo[33] wrote a Twitter thread called "Is it gender bias, or do I just suck?" describing several situations in which she (or someone she knows) experienced gender bias. Because it is more subtle than overt discrimination or harassment, trainees may not think it is worth reporting. Finally, it is difficult to know how to respond to bias with no clear reporting structure.

Trainees should document biased comments or behavior, including the time, place, and quote direct statements. They should also keep any documented evidence of bias, such as emails, texts, or photos. Trainees should identify an ally to whom they can report the incident or behavior. The person could be a faculty whom the trainee trusts, the program director, or the designated ombudsperson by the training program and affiliated department of human resources. On the part of the residency program, protocols should be in place to deal with incoming complaints or concerns of unfair treatment. These should also be aligned with protocols at the institutional level for all graduate medical educational programs. Depending on the situation, the goal of reporting may vary from awareness to apology to remediation to punishment. Trainees should also build support networks, inside and outside of the residency program. Sharing stories about bias and how to respond to it helps decrease the mental toll that bias can take over time.

Teaching about UB is no easy task. Many schools have incorporated the IAT as a standard assessment for incoming medical students; however, putting the results to good use requires commitment and more than a single intervention. A study by Gonzalez and colleagues[34] suggests that a single session is insufficient to offer adequate instruction on UB. In their study, 22% of students surveyed actually denied the results of their IAT. When done properly, however, the results are rewarding. A follow-up study highlighted the importance of longitudinal training for a UB curriculum.[35] The study by Geller and Watkins[11] reported that up to 30% of students described improvements in their attitudes following ethics training aimed at influencing their weight-based biases. Thus, in developing UB education, a longitudinal curriculum should be emphasized as opposed to haphazard or ad hoc sessions.

Targeted Strategies for Faculty

The issues of UB among faculty are even more challenging because they must be managed and addressed in different domains including interactions with trainees, peers, and those that may affect patient care. As academic and clinical leaders, surgical faculty are well positioned to eliminate UB in surgical education. Faculty awareness of concepts of UB can make equitable matriculation into surgical residency. In addition, as surgical leaders transition from early career to midcareer and advanced career faculty, new responsibilities include faculty mentorship, sponsorship, and coaching.

To be a successful mentor, sponsor, or academic coach, an individual does not need to look like the colleague they are helping. When midcareer and senior faculty who are not of color are to mentor, sponsor, or coach colleagues of color, or colleagues who are not of the same gender, they should understand and acknowledge that particular colleague's professional needs. These may include professional development training, access to opportunities and networks, emotional support to manage the stressors of academic advancement, institutional sponsorship, role models whose success they want to emulate, safe spaces to discuss experiences, and honest constructive feedback.[36] In addition, if an individual cannot directly mentor their early career colleagues, then that individual's professional expertise can still be of value. They can direct their diverse junior faculty colleagues to other faculty members who can fulfill their individual mentoring needs, forming a mentoring team.

Faculty are uniquely positioned to improve the resident selection process by understanding their own UB and acknowledging the multiple layers in an applicant's journey. This includes selection for honors societies, letters of recommendation, and applicant selection. "Blind spots" in cultural awareness are counterproductive to effective faculty leadership. Santen and colleagues[37] queried fourth-year medical students from a single medical school after the residency match. A total of 90% of the students were asked at least one potentially discriminatory question, including questions about their marital status, about children, family planning, nationality, and religious beliefs.

A solution is to implement standardized interview questions that are germane to what the trainee may experience at the residency program, with a scoring system grading the interviews response to the questions, as opposed to a free-flowing unstructured interview.[38] Because few residency programs currently use structured interviews, this is an opportunity for innovation in cardiothoracic surgery education.[39,40]

Several academic institutions are leading the way in local efforts to increase URM retention, productivity, and promotion. A small subset have conducted prospective studies demonstrating effectiveness of their programs boasting increases in faculty retention, promotion, and representation of up to 80% to 90%.[41,42] Similarly, interventions aimed at improving gender bias among faculty have also shown some success. The University of Wisconsin sought to address gender bias among its faculty within 92 departments or divisions using a cluster randomized control study. The experimental departments were subjected to a 2.5-hour workshop on gender bias intervention. The authors reported significantly greater changes postintervention for faculty in experimental versus control departments on several outcome measures, including self-efficacy to engage in gender-equity-promoting behaviors. When greater than or equal to 25% of a department's faculty attended the workshop, significant increases in self-reported action to promote gender equity occurred at 3 months. Postintervention, faculty in experimental departments expressed greater perceptions of fit, valuing of their research, and comfort in raising personal and professional conflicts.[43]

Targeted Strategies for the Institution

As an institution, with the full support of leadership at all levels, a commitment to the principles of diversity and inclusion by striving to create a culture in which all students, faculty, and staff feel respected and valued is a must. Recruiting and retaining a diverse community and creating a climate of respect that is supportive of their success encourages innovation and enhances a department's ability to fulfill its core mission: inclusive excellence.

Regular programming managed by human resources personnel and/or the school of medicine serves to establish a culture of inclusion and a sense of collaboration, trust, and zero tolerance for overt bias and microaggressions. Some organizations have incorporated the IAT into various facets of training and leadership. UB is a habit that is remediated through literacy training and education to reduce discrimination. Institutions must also empower residents, faculty, and staff to report discriminatory practices without fear of retaliation or retribution. Addressing issues of UB and overt bias at the institutional level requires not only acknowledgment that these issues exist and persist in modern health care environments, but also that they undermine the academic mission of institutions.

Specific efforts to create a more inclusive and diverse health care environment starts with a well-articulated vision by senior leadership on a regular and consistent basis (**Box 3**). This vision should clearly outline the benefits of such a program for the entire health care organization and emphasize it as a core value in the vision statement.

It is evident that if an organization is developing such a vision as a new focus or emphasis, it takes time to change a culture that otherwise has not focused on these issues previously. It is hoped this is a "proactive" emphasis, rather than a "reactive" approach to addressing ongoing concerns or issues.

Leadership development and environmental change

Leadership development in the areas of diversity and inclusion not only raises awareness about the problems of UB but also endeavors to develop leaders from the majority and underrepresented health care communities to affect change in the health care environment. In an ideal institutionally supported environment, these programs are the responsibility of the majority and the URM. Dedicated leadership development programming and instruction are necessary to enhance the change in culture of these environments. The responsibility for these diversity programs often falls to the diversity and inclusion institutional official appointed either in the school of medicine as a dean or health system vice president as the "accountable leader." In addition, many URMs are often recruited to participate in the programming related to these issues; the so called "minority tax."

It is a collective responsibility of the academic and surgical leadership and all surgical faculty in an educational program to enhance diversity and change the culture of the environment to be more inclusive. Underrepresented minority students, residents and faculty can and should serve as ambassadors for diversity. Leadership and faculty development are further advanced by systematic training at the institutional and association level. The American College of Surgeons, the

---

Box 3
Representative vision and goals statements

- Increase faculty, student, and staff diversity through broad recruitment, training engagement, and retention efforts
- Creation of a more inclusive academic environment by enhancing transparency and accountability for all members of the health care environment

American Heart Association, the American Association of Thoracic Surgery, the Society of Thoracic Surgeons, Women in Thoracic Surgery, the National Institutes of Health Minority Access to Research Careers program, and several other professional organizations have developed leadership programs to address diversity and inclusion. The Society of Black Academic Surgeons Leadership and Faculty Development Institute was developed in 2006 to provide intense and focused leadership training and mentorship for minority academic surgeons. These programs enhance the skill sets of future leaders through a variety of program elements focusing on mentorship, strategic planning, conflict resolution, and the value of sponsorship.

Our primary aim is to provide a framework that outlines strategies and skills that can be taught to medical trainees and practicing physicians, to prevent unconscious attitudes and stereotypes from negatively influencing the course and outcomes of clinical encounters. These strategies and skills are designed to (1) enhance internal motivation to reduce bias, while avoiding external pressure; (2) increase understanding about the psychological basis of bias; (3) enhance providers' confidence in their ability to successfully interact with socially dissimilar patients; (4) enhance emotional regulation skills; and (5) improve the ability to build partnerships with patients.[44,45]

SUMMARY

UB is ubiquitous and affects our daily lives and work. Cardiothoracic surgery is no exception to its influence. Most often used for creating mental shortcuts, it can also influence the way in which we support and select medical students and residents for training, how and what we teach the trainee, and how we may inadvertently perpetuate disparities in care and diversity within our workforce. Once we acknowledge the presence of UB, we will be successful in implementing strategies to mitigate its negative influence. "Extraordinary people are not extraordinary because they are invulnerable to unconscious biases. They are extraordinary because they choose to do something about it" (Shankar Vedantam).[46]

REFERENCES

1. Fiarman S. Unconscious bias: when good intentions aren't enough. Disrupting Inequity 2016; 74(3):10–5.
2. Frank MC, Vul E, Johnson SP. Development of infants' attention to faces during the first year. Cognition 2009;110(2):160–70.
3. Antonoff MB, David EA, Donington JS, et al. Women in thoracic surgery: 30 years of history. Ann Thorac Surg 2016;101(1):399–409.
4. Abelson JS, Symer MM, Yeo HL, et al. Surgical time out: our counts are still short on racial diversity in academic surgery. Am J Surg 2018;215(4):542–8.
5. Correll J, Park B, Judd CM, et al. Across the thin blue line: police officers and racial bias in the decision to shoot. J Pers Soc Psychol 2007;92(6):1006–23.
6. Green AR, Carney DR, Pallin DJ, et al. Implicit bias among physicians and its prediction of thrombolysis decisions for black and white patients. J Gen Intern Med 2007;22(9):1231–8.
7. Ruck MD, Tenenbaum HR, Sines J. Brief report: British adolescents' views about the rights of asylum-seeking children. J Adolesc 2007;30(4):687–93.
8. Greenwald AG, McGhee DE, Schwartz JL. Measuring individual differences in implicit cognition: the implicit association test. J Pers Soc Psychol 1998;74(6):1464–80.
9. Capers QT, Clinchot D, McDougle L, et al. Implicit racial bias in medical school admissions. Acad Med 2017;92(3):365–9.
10. van Ryn M, Hardeman RR, Phelan SM, et al. Psychosocial predictors of attitudes toward physician empathy in clinical encounters among 4732 1st year medical students: a report from the CHANGES study. Patient Educ Couns 2014;96(3):367–75.
11. Geller G, Watkins PA. Addressing medical students' negative bias toward patients with obesity through ethics education. AMA J Ethics 2018;20(10):E948–59.
12. Institute of Medicine Committee on U, Eliminating R, Ethnic Disparities in Health C. In: Smedley BD, Stith AY, Nelson AR, editors. Unequal treatment: confronting racial and ethnic disparities in health care. Washington (DC): National Academies Press (US); 2003. Copyright 2002 by the National Academy of Sciences. All rights reserved.
13. Meza JM, Rectenwald JE, Reddy RM. The bias against integrated thoracic surgery residency applicants during general surgery interviews. Ann Thorac Surg 2015;99(4):1206–12.
14. Falcone JL. Home-field advantage: the role of selection bias in the general surgery national residency matching program. J Surg Educ 2013;70(4):461–5.
15. Gerull KM, Loe M, Seiler K, et al. Assessing gender bias in qualitative evaluations of surgical residents. Am J Surg 2019;217(2):306–13.
16. Phillips NA, Tannan SC, Kalliainen LK. Understanding and overcoming implicit gender bias in plastic surgery. Plast Reconstr Surg 2016;138(5):1111–6.
17. Dresler CM, Padgett DL, MacKinnon SE, et al. Experiences of women in cardiothoracic surgery. A gender comparison. Arch Surg 1996;131(11): 1128–34 [discussion: 1135].
18. Bruce AN, Battista A, Plankey MW, et al. Perceptions of gender-based discrimination during surgical

training and practice. Med Educ Online 2015;20: 25923.

19. Myers SP, Hill KA, Nicholson KJ, et al. A qualitative study of gender differences in the experiences of general surgery trainees. J Surg Res 2018;228:127–34.

20. Wong RL, Sullivan MC, Yeo HL, et al. Race and surgical residency: results from a national survey of 4339 US general surgery residents. Ann Surg 2013;257(4):782–7.

21. Dayal A, O'Connor DM, Qadri U, et al. Comparison of male vs female resident milestone evaluations by faculty during emergency medicine residency training. JAMA Intern Med 2017;177(5): 651–7.

22. Mueller AS, Jenkins TM, Osborne M, et al. Gender differences in attending physicians' feedback to residents: a qualitative analysis. J Grad Med Educ 2017;9(5):577–05.

23. Salles A, Mueller CM, Cohen GL. A values affirmation intervention to improve female residents' surgical performance. J Grad Med Educ 2016;8(3): 378–83.

24. Meyerson SL, Sternbach JM, Zwischenberger JB, et al. The effect of gender on resident autonomy in the operating room. J Surg Educ 2017;74(6):e111–8.

25. Thompson-Burdine J, Sutzko DC, Nikolian VC, et al. Impact of a resident's sex on intraoperative entrustment of surgery trainees. Surgery 2018;164(3):583–8.

26. Stephens EH, Robich MP, Walters DM, et al. Gender and cardiothoracic surgery training: specialty interests, satisfaction, and career pathways. Ann Thorac Surg 2016;102(1):200–6.

27. Rodriguez JE, Campbell KM, Fogarty JP, et al. Underrepresented minority faculty in academic medicine: a systematic review of URM faculty development. Fam Med 2014;46(2):100–4.

28. Abelson JS, Wong NZ, Symer M, et al. Racial and ethnic disparities in promotion and retention of academic surgeons. Am J Surg 2018;216(4): 678–82.

29. Files JA, Mayer AP, Ko MG, et al. Speaker introductions at internal medicine grand rounds: forms of address reveal gender bias. J Womens Health (Larchmt) 2017;26(5):413–9.

30. Fassiotto M, Li J, Maldonado Y, et al. Female surgeons as counter stereotype: the impact of gender perceptions on trainee evaluations of physician faculty. J Surg Educ 2018;75(5):1140–8.

31. Sarsons H. Interpreting signals in the labor market: evidence from medical referrals [Job Market Paper]. In.

32. Osseo-Asare A, Balasuriya L, Huot SJ, et al. Minority resident physicians' views on the role of race/ethnicity in their training experiences in the workplace. JAMA Netw Open 2018;1(5):e182723.

33. Choo E. Is it gender bias, or do I just suck?. 2018. Available at: https://twitter.com/choo_ek. Accessed March 1, 2018.

34. Gonzalez CM, Kim MY, Marantz PR. Implicit bias and its relation to health disparities: a teaching program and survey of medical students. Teach Learn Med 2014;26(1):64–71.

35. Gonzalez CM, Garba RJ, Liguori A, et al. How to make or break implicit bias instruction: implications for curriculum development. Acad Med 2018;93:S74–81 (11S Association of American Medical Colleges Learn Serve Lead: Proceedings of the 57th Annual Research in Medical Education Sessions).

36. KA R. Can I mentor African-American faculty? 2016. Available at: https://www.insidehighered.com/advice/2016/02/17/advice-white-professor-about-mentoring-scholars-color-essay. Accessed November 24, 2018.

37. Santen SA, Davis KR, Brady DW, et al. Potentially discriminatory questions during residency interviews: frequency and effects on residents' ranking of programs in the national resident matching program. J Grad Med Educ 2010;2(3):336–40.

38. Huffcutt AI. From science to practice: seven principles for conducting employment interviews. Appl H R M Res 2010;12(1):121–36.

39. Kim RH, Gilbert T, Suh S, et al. General surgery residency interviews: are we following best practices? Am J Surg 2016;211(2):476–81.e3.

40. Whitgob EE, Blankenburg RL, Bogetz AL. The discriminatory patient and family: strategies to address discrimination towards trainees. Acad Med 2016;91:S64–9 (11 Association of American Medical Colleges Learn Serve Lead: Proceedings of the 55th Annual research in medical education sessions).

41. Wingard D, Trejo J, Gudea M, et al. Faculty equity, diversity, culture and climate change in academic medicine: a longitudinal study. J Natl Med Assoc 2019;111(1):16–53.

42. Deas D, Pisano ED, Mainous AG, et al. Improving diversity through strategic planning: a 10-year (2002-2012) experience at the Medical University of South Carolina. Acad Med 2012;87(11): 1548–55.

43. Carnes M, Devine PG, Baier Manwell L, et al. The effect of an intervention to break the gender bias habit for faculty at one institution: a cluster randomized, controlled trial. Acad Med 2015;90(2):221–30.

44. Burgess D, van Ryn M, Dovidio J, et al. Reducing racial bias among health care providers: lessons from social-cognitive psychology. J Gen Intern Med 2007;22(6):882–7.

45. Glicksman E. Unconscious bias in academic medicine: overcoming the prejudices we don't know we have [press release]. AAMC2016.

46. Vedantam S. The hidden brain: how our unconscious minds elect presidents, control markets, wage wars, and save our lives. 1st edition. New York: Spiegel & Grau; 2010.

Educational Challenges of the Operating Room

Christopher R. Morse, MD*, Douglas J. Mathisen, MD

KEYWORDS

- Operative education • Operative teaching • Intraoperative education • Surgeon educator

KEY POINTS

- Complexity in cardiothoracic (CT) surgery continues to increase with incoming CT residents having varying degrees of exposure before starting fellowship.
- External factors such as public reporting and a push for increased case volume continue to influence the willingness of attending surgeons to involve residents in operative cases.
- Opportunities to improve the operative education experience have never been more diverse including a comprehensive curriculum, simulations, and educational "boot camps."

Resident education in the operating room and surgical resident autonomy represent 2 enormous challenges within cardiothoracic (CT) training programs. The goal of surgical educators and CT trainees is to ensure the graduating resident's ability to safely operate independently at the completion of training. The field has come a long way from the notion of see one, do one, teach one, which was once the norm. CT surgery continues to become more specialized and the patients more complex with greater scrutiny of outcomes. The need to integrate technological advances comes at a rapid pace. There are many challenges that are faced in contemporary CT training to make intraoperative teaching harder than ever (**Box 1**). Often unspoken is the importance of having a mindset dedicated to taking residents through operations, allowing them to make intraoperative decisions and developing autonomy. Some possess this mindset and others struggle with the concept of giving portions of the operation away.

EXTERNAL FORCES

The operating room remains the pinnacle of experiential learning but remains the least structured of all educational activities during surgical training.

CT surgery has changed enormously over the last 35 years. In 1982, the cases recorded for the American Board of Thoracic Surgery (ABTS) for a graduating thoracic track resident from a 1-year program are seen in **Table 1**. This is compared with the current cases reported to the ABTS for a two-and-a-half–year training program for a thoracic track resident. The total experience gained over more time is currently much greater, but the experience comes much later because of less experience coming into fellowship training. The amount of time spent on CT rotations before entering fellowship training has dramatically changed. Residents 30 years ago had much more exposure to cardiac and thoracic surgery as a general surgery resident, often times 12 to 16 months for cardiac surgery and 4 to 6 months for general thoracic surgery during 5 years of general surgery training. Currently residents spend between 2 and 6 months on cardiac surgery, the most common being 2 months spent in the cardiac intensive care unit as a second-year resident. Thoracic surgery rotations are generally available as an intern and fourth year resident totaling 4 months. Very few general surgery training programs provide senior level rotations on cardiac surgery. Therefore, residents come in less

Disclosure Statement: The authors have nothing to disclose.
Thoracic Surgery, Massachusetts General Hospital, 55 Fruit Street, FND 7, Boston, MA 02114, USA
* Corresponding author.
E-mail address: crmorse@partners.org

Thorac Surg Clin 29 (2019) 269–277
https://doi.org/10.1016/j.thorsurg.2019.03.005

Box 1
Current challenges to operative teaching

1. Less time in cardiothoracic surgery during general surgery training
2. Less time in associated fields and less open surgery (vascular surgery)
3. Loss of preoperative day
4. Older, sicker, more complex patients, case mix
5. Work hours—resident autonomy
6. Measuring outcomes and public reporting and medical malpractice
7. Hospital pressure to increase productivity, reduce costs and length of stay, and improve outcomes
8. Greater emphasis on surgeon productivity generating relative value units tied to reimbursement
9. Transition to practice and rapidly evolving technology

prepared for CT training. Another factor is the loss of a preoperative day, which has had the unintended consequences of residents being less acquainted with patients and their surgical problems. This means less opportunity to examine the patient, review important and pertinent

Table 1
Operative experience of a thoracic track resident

	1982 (1 y)	2014 (2.5 y)
	Cardiac (4 mo)	Cardiac (12 mo)
Valve	34	27
CABG	47	55
Aorta	0	5
Congenital	9	3
Transplant	0	21
Total	90	111
	Thoracic (7 mo)	Thoracic (16 mo)
Lung	79	258 (26 VATS)
Esophagus	28	109 (22 MIE)
Airway	5	16
Total	112	283
Combined	202	394

Abbreviations: CABG, coronary artery bypass surgery; MIE, minimally invasive esophagectomy; VATS, video-assisted thoracic surgery.

studies, and correlate these studies with their physical examination and history. Residents often meet the patient on the day of surgery in the operating room; this allows for less preparation for the operation and puts an extra burden on the resident and the attending surgeon. The case mix available for training has also dramatically changed. Thirty years ago, there were an abundance of straightforward coronary artery bypass surgeries, valves, and more straightforward congenital heart surgery procedures. There were no stents, extracorporeal membrane oxygenations, ventricular assist devices, neoadjuvant therapy, or minimally invasive procedures to complicate matters and make introduction to basic cardiac and thoracic surgery more challenging. Many of the currently available cases are not appropriate for beginning CT residents.

EXTERNAL FORCES AFFECTING THE TEACHING ENVIRONMENT

The threat of medical malpractice is real, and although unspoken, influences resident involvement in operations. Concern over complications and bad outcomes may lead to less operative experience for residents. Cardiac surgery and thoracic surgery are highly scrutinized by hospital, payers, and the government. The Society of Thoracic Surgeons database allows extensive data collection on each procedure. Outcomes are analyzed with highly accurate data for the individual surgeon and collectively the surgical group. Programs are ranked based on their risk-adjusted outcomes. The outcomes by surgical groups are now publicly reported for cardiac surgery and increasingly so for thoracic surgery. Individual surgeon reporting is soon to become the norm. This policy can lead to "risk averse behavior" and influence the willingness of attending surgeons to involve residents in operative cases and a loss of experience. Cost of health care is another not so subtle factor influencing surgical training. Hospital budgets continue to be under pressure. There is a tremendous emphasis to increase productivity and reduce costs and a focus on operative times, utilization of resources, and length of stay. Some studies have shown increased operative times with resident involvement, thereby increasing cost and decreasing efficiency.[1–3] There are well-recognized data on the impact of complications related to cost.[4,5] There are conflicting data on the influence of resident participation on outcomes, but some studies suggest that with careful supervision the impact is little different, whether the procedure is done by attending surgeon or resident.[6,7] Medicare has mandated no payment for complications for "never events." Mediastinitis is one of the "never events," thereby increasing the emphasis on avoiding complications and indirectly affecting resident training.[8] Currently Medicare and most payers now demand attending surgeon's presence for "the critical part of operations" and strict rules about avoidance of concurrent surgery. These policies have as their rationale patient safety and improved outcomes. These principles are important but clearly have indirect or direct impact on resident autonomy and training.

Increasingly physician reimbursement is tied to productivity, generation of "RVUs," and employment by hospitals. With increasing numbers of surgeons employed by hospitals, productivity and outcomes are closely monitored and measured. These factors subtly influence resident teaching. There is greater pressure to do more in less time, reduce costs, avoid complications, and improve outcomes. This trend may lead to greater reluctance to involve residents.

WORK HOURS

In 2002, the ACGME instituted work hour restrictions (before this standard, it was not uncommon for residents to work up to 120 hours per week). An excellent analysis of the impact of reducing resident work hours to 80 hours has been presented by Lewis and colleagues[9] (**Box 2**). Going from 100 to 80 hours reduces the overall clinical training in a 5-year general surgery program by 1 year. Reducing work hours from 90 to 80 results in reduction of one and a half years of clinical exposure. Little attention has been paid to address this loss of clinical exposure. These are not just theoretic considerations. Connors and

colleagues[10] conducted a retrospective study of 4 CT training programs in the Western United States. This study looked at the impact of the implementation of work hours on cases reported to the ABTS before and after the introduction of work hour restrictions (**Table 2**). A reduction in overall operative experience in cardiac surgery was identified. There was not a corresponding reduction in surgical experience for thoracic surgical cases. Few studies have been done since this report and whether this trend has continued or not is important information but currently not known. More subtle impact of work hour restrictions are loss of autonomy, doing cases when on call, requiring residents to leave the hospital after being on call leading to missed operative cases, and less time to prepare and review patients' records.[11]

PROFESSION'S RESPONSE TO CHALLENGES OF OPERATIVE TEACHING

Around the year 2000, ABTS identified a dramatic decline in the interest of general surgery residents in CT training. This dramatic decline led to a situation where there were a fewer applicants than positions available. The profession recognized that it must act quickly, decisively, and reverse this trend (**Box 3**). It was clear that the specialty had taken for granted resident interest. The first action taken by ABTS was to eliminate the requirement for American Board of Surgery certification. This was done in the hope to reduce overall length of training and create opportunities for new training paradigms. The integrated 6-year program (I-6) and the integrated General Surgery Cardiothoracic (4/3) pathways into CT surgery training were created. This was done in the hopes of stimulating interest in the specialty. There are currently about thirty I-6 and fifteen 4/3 programs. The I-6 program has mostly been emphasized in cardiac surgery and the 4/3 for those more broadly interested in

---

Box 2
Impact of reduction of resident work hours on clinical time

Before 2003

  100 h/wk = 48 wk × 5 y = 24,000 h

  90 h/wk = 48 wk × 5 y = 21,600 h

  80 h/wk = 48 wk × 5 y = 19,200 h

100 to 80 = 4800 h reduction = 1 y equivalent

90 to 80 = 2400 h reduction = 0.5 y equivalent

Overall impact: 10% to 20% reduction in clinical time

No corresponding adjustments

Data from Lewis FR, Klingensmith ME. Issues in general surgery residency training. Ann Surg 2012;256:55–9.

Table 2
Effect of work hour restriction on operative experience in cardiothoracic surgical training

Year	Cardiac Cases		P Value
	Before 80-h Limit	After 80-h Limit	
1	190	153	.15
2	154	108	<.0001
3	115	75	.001

Data from Connors RC, Doty JR, Bull DA, et al. Effect of work-hour restriction on operative experience in cardiothoracic surgical residency training. J Thorac Cardiovasc Surg 2009;137:710–3.

Box 3
Profession's response to challenges of operative teaching

1. Creation of I-6 and 4/3 training paradigms

2. Web-based CT curriculum

3. EACTS multimedia project

4. Simulation, both operative and situational (cardiopulmonary bypass)

5. TSDA Boot Camp, Top Gun Program

6. Educate the Educator courses

7. Development of the time-out checklist

8. Tools to evaluate performance, SIMPL, ZWISCH, and PASS

9. Development of "How I Teach It" topics in The Annals of Thoracic Surgery

10. Milestone project

Abbreviation: TSDA, Thoracic Surgery Directors' Association.

CT surgery. These changes have been a major factor in stimulating interest, with the current ratio of applicants to positions being 1.5:1, up from .75:1 ten years ago! These training programs allow earlier exposure to the specialty and more gradual introduction to the care and surgery of CT patients.

Along with the redesign of the training programs was a major emphasis on teaching and education. An interactive, web-based curriculum has been adopted by all CT training programs with access to a vast array of written materials and instructive videos. The European Association of Cardiothoracic Surgery has developed a complementary "Multimedia Journal" that features operative videos from acclaimed experts. These platforms allow easy access to review all aspects of operations: evaluation, indications, operative approach, technical details, and management of complications. Residents are able to access this information before going to the operating room and prepare for the conduct of specific operations.

Models were created that allowed deliberate practice with careful supervision done in a nonstressful setting. Animal organs were used to create a nearly lifelike simulation for tactile sense of the tissues and what it was like to operate on CT organs. Most operations in CT surgery can be replicated. With attending supervision, very specific details can be stressed during the course of simulated operations. Time is not a factor, and direct supervision is allowed for precision, proficiency, and understanding. Simulation programs were developed at the national meetings such as "Top Gun" where a competition was held between

residents to measure their technical proficiency. Speed and accuracy were the metrics that were measured. This activity energized future and current residents. Low-fidelity models were developed that allowed deliberate practice away from the hospital. Practical models were developed, which allowed suturing with magnification, cardiac instrumentation, and fine sutures. These models also allowed for videotaping, longitudinal assessment, and deliberate practice. Situational simulation was also developed. These situational efforts mimic real-life situations in the operating room. The most effective models were those developed for the conduct of cardiopulmonary bypass. Various scenarios could be created where emergencies arose and subsequent understanding of how to manage them. Such a course has been given annually at the Society of Thoracic Surgeons. They have been very valuable in teaching real situations in a controlled environment. Team work simulation was also developed and had an indirect impact on operative teaching.

The Thoracic Surgery Directors' Association developed the "CT Resident Boot Camp." This has been a very successful program that stresses simulation. It is designed for CT residents and junior faculty. Models of many cardiac and thoracic procedures are available for simulation. The residents and junior faculty are introduced to the principles and opportunity with surgical simulation. At present every training program has had at least one faculty member participate and hundreds of residents. No one thinks a single introduction to simulation will improve performance, but with repetitive, deliberate practice, this can accelerate a resident's technical expertise. This concept of repetitive, deliberate practice introduced by Ericsson and others[12,13] has been widely adopted. To that end, the ABTS now requires 20 hours of documented simulation experience for CT residents. Simulation is not a substitute for operative experience, but it can accelerate the learning curve. Properly organized and staffed, it greatly aids intraoperative teaching.

To improve the educators' teaching abilities, courses were developed to "educate the educators." At the present time every training program in America has had representatives attend these courses. Networking, educational theory, and hands-on and situational simulation are stressed. It is hoped that each individual will incorporate their experience into improved teaching in their training program.

Many other programs were developed, indirectly related to operative teaching. The creation of timeout checklists was promulgated and is used in most operating rooms around the United

States. This concept allows for greater awareness of the operation, the procedure, instrumentation, and anticipated problems, thereby reducing overall stress and allowing a better environment in which to work. This is followed by a similar checklist at the end of the procedure to go through parts of the operation, identify concerns, and raise general awareness.[14] Educational tools have been created to evaluate intraoperative resident performance including several smartphone applications.[15,16] These tools allow immediate assessment of a resident's performance and provide feedback immediately after the completion of an operation. This informs the resident of their operative performance and progress as well as areas for improvement.

The Annals of Thoracic Surgery has created a special section on "How I Teach It." These are specific operations described in great detail by recognized experts in the field.[17] This feature has been well received. These contributions are geared specifically to teach the procedure and are valuable for young attendings interested in surgical teaching.

Finally, the Accreditation Council for Graduate Medical Education has developed the milestone project, which is designed to create a regular evaluation of a resident's progress during the course of their residency (**Box 4**). Every 6 months residents are evaluated by a group of attending surgeons and a checklist is created allowing systematic evaluation of the resident's performance in a variety of areas. The hope is that over time progress will be identified and residents will improve and go from novice to expert. It is hoped that at the end of the training program all residents move to the expert category. This competency-based approach to surgery has great merit but is in its infancy. The day has not come in cardiac and thoracic surgery where residents are allowed to finish training based on their competence, rather still a fixed number of operations and a specified period of training are required.

EXPECTATIONS OF ATTENDING SENIOR SURGEON AND RESIDENT

There are expectations of the senior surgeon and resident for every operation (**Table 3**). There are certain expectations of both the attending senior surgeon and resident. The conduct of each operation begins with preparation. The senior surgeon is the one in charge. This individual must be prepared, be able to manage his or her stress, and guarantee a safe, successful outcome of the operation at the same time guiding residents through appropriate cases. For the attending surgeon, this begins with preparation and deep understanding of the problem and the operation that is to be carried out. Operative stress is managed by preparation; the better the preparation, the lesser the stress; the lesser the stress, the better the learning environment. Communication is an important part of the operative experience and teaching. All levels of the health care team, nurses, anesthesiologist, and residents must be involved in open and specific communication, so that everyone is on the same page. There should be no surprises during the course of an operation except those that are unexpected. Various methods have been developed to enhance this aspect of surgical teaching such as time-outs, preoperative huddles, and checklists. It is incumbent on the attending surgeon to review the details with the resident of each case: radiographs, data, and cath results. The resident should be expected to "know" the patient if they are going to participate in the case. The attending surgeon must be available for every step of the operation the resident is uncertain about. This might start with the skin incision and end with the skin closure and all steps in between. The more senior surgical residents may have greater autonomy during various steps of the operation, but this should be determined by the attending surgeon and agreed to by the resident. The resident should not be put in any uncomfortable situation for which they are not prepared or experienced. The attending surgeon should stress technical details despite the previous experience of the resident. CT surgery for many is a new experience. Although the resident may have skills developed during general surgery, they may not be directly applicable to CT surgery. Anticoagulation, different instruments, fine suture material, and the need for magnification are all things that should be emphasized by the attending surgeon. Basic details should be stressed: how to hold the needle holder, the angle of the needle, how to comfortably position oneself at the operating table, and ways to reduce tremors. The attending surgeon should stress the conduct of the operation to the resident surgeon. How to go from point A to point B, from point B to point C, and from point C to point F if a change in plans is required is not necessarily intuitive for most CT residents. It is helpful to talk out loud and identify

Box 4
Example of milestones in cardiac surgery

Level I	Do sternotomy
Level II	Cannulating
Level III	Take-down of the mammary
Level IV	Routine coronary bypass
Level V	Redo coronary artery bypass

Table 3
Operative expectations of senior surgeon and resident

Senior Surgeon	Resident
1. Preparation each case	1. Come prepared about patient and operation
2. Communicate to OR team, especially resident	2. Practice–simulation–deliberate practice. Review steps of operation
3. Review details of case (cath, radiographs) and approach with resident	3. Ask questions of surgeon, ask to review cath, radiographs, data
4. Be available for every step resident is uncertain of	4. Intense focus/concentration on technique and steps of operation
5. Stress technical details, holding needle holder, where to place the stitches	5. Strive for perfection
6. Stress conduct of operation A to B, B to C, etc., and alternate ways to proceed	6. Debrief, ask about expectations and concerns
7. Identify "pitfalls" how to avoid and manage	7. Accept constructive criticism
8. At all times, stress perfection	8. Personal debrief details of case, tricks/tips, take notes
9. Identify postop concerns and how to manage	9. Understand entrustment
10. Develop "entrustment"	10. Develop "grit"
11. Develop "grit"	

potential pitfalls at every step of the operation, how to be aware of them, and how to manage them if problems develop. At all times of the operation, it is important to stress perfection. Vince Lombardi, the famous coach of the Green Bay Packers, is quoted as saying "Perfection is not attainable, but if we chase perfection we can catch excellence."[18] This concept applies to surgery as well. On completion of the operation, the attending surgeon should express their concerns—potential problems that may develop and how to identify and manage them—which should be discussed with the resident and passed along to the intensive care team. At all steps of the operation, patient safety is paramount.

Autonomy has become a big issue in surgical education. Both the senior surgeon and the resident must understand the concept of "entrustment," whereby responsibility is given to the resident or appropriate autonomy granted during the course of the operation. Five levels of entrustment have been identified by Cate and colleagues[19]: level 1, no independence; level 2, close supervision; level 3, limited supervision; level 4, act independently; and level 5, supervise others. The current regulations of medicine make it very difficult to allow independent operation by residents. However, the safest operation is one done with an attending surgeon and resident, whereby the resident has satisfied all expectations and is allowed to perform the operation under the watchful eye and careful supervision of the attending

surgeon. The highest degree of autonomy that can be achieved and the safest experience for the patient is where a resident places every stitch and the attending says not a single word during the operation because the resident has done them perfectly. Oftentimes residents equate autonomy or entrustment with independent operation without the presence of an attending surgeon. When done right, every stitch is an autonomous event, with the safeguard of a senior surgeon to confirm it has been done perfectly.

EXPECTATIONS OF THE TRAINEE

It should be expected of every resident that they come prepared to the operating room. The burden is on the residents to do this on their own before the operation. They may not have met the patient before surgery, but they are expected to have reviewed all the data, radiographs, cath reports, and physiologic data and understand the patient's problem and the operation to be performed. Before coming to the operating room, they should avail themselves of any simulation opportunity to practice the operation or to practice various components of the operation such as performing the anastomosis, using loupes, special needle holders, and fine suture material. The resident should review the various steps of the operation. They should watch videos if available. They should read descriptions of the operation so that they are well informed. They should not be hesitant to ask questions of the surgeon to explore what were the indications for surgery and how they chose to perform the planned operation. At all times the resident should ask the attending about various parts of an operation for clarification. Residents must develop the ability for intense focus and concentration. They must apply this intense concentration to every technical detail and step of the operation. The resident must also strive for perfection. Although at first this may be a faraway goal, with practice and repetition, they will get closer to achieving this goal. At the end of an operation there should be a debriefing about what was done, what is expected of the patient, what pitfalls and problems might occur, and how to identify and manage them. Each resident should personally debrief themselves regarding their conduct of the operation and the operation itself. They should learn how to take constructive criticism, whether it is through direct communication or the use of one of the many tools now available to evaluate resident performance and provide feedback.

Angela Duckworth,[20] a cognitive psychologist, advanced the concept of "GRIT." She describes this as being essential to performance at the highest levels. Her book, "Grit: The Power of Passion and Perseverance," defines this concept. She defines grit as the positive noncognitive trait based on an individual's passion for a particular long-term goal or end state coupled with a powerful motivation to achieve that objective. The perseverance of effort promotes overcoming the obstacles or challenges that line an individual's path to accomplishment and serves as a driving force and achievement realization. Grit has 2 fundamental components, consistency of interest and perseverance of effort. She believes that this concept of "grit" is an important individual character trait capable of predicting long-term success. How does this apply in the operating room? There are many stressful, unexpected events that occur in highly demanding operations. One must develop the ability to deal with these situations, manage stress, persevere to get the best outcome for each patient, and develop this trait of "GRIT." This is important for the senior surgeon to possess and the resident to develop. When in a difficult situation, the surgeon must keep operating!

FUTURE SOLUTIONS

The authors have identified many challenges in operative teaching. Some are technical, some are situational, and some are educational. The future relies on many of the basic tools that are available today (**Box 5**). The authors have stressed the importance of simulation, preparation, and

---

> **Box 5**
> **Future solutions**
>
> 1. Three-dimensional printing to clearly define complex anatomy
> 2. Improved computer simulation to replicate operations
> 3. Robots and robotics to improve outcomes
> 4. Improved instrumentation
> 5. Early exposure I-6/4/3 programs
> 6. Apprentice model—works if exposed broadly to surgeons and breadth of specialty. Challenging for 4/3 thoracic track residents in cardiac surgery

becoming better at what they do. Simulation will also evolve to allow simulation of entire operations, either on computer-based platforms or the use of lifelike models. Three-dimensional (3D) printing has entered CT surgery. The ability to 3D print very complicated anatomy, complicated congenital anomalies, or extensive tumors so that this can be reviewed and understood before the conduct of the operation is an exciting prospect. 3D printing may allow individuals to actually perform an operation in the wet laboratory before the operating room. Robots and robotics will continue to evolve and become a bigger part of CT surgery. Precision that can be achieved with robotics should lead to better outcomes. Visualization will be enhanced, and experience will be acquired by those devoted to miniaturizing operations. Improved instrumentation will be needed for all types of minimally invasive surgery. Advances in haptic recognition will improve robotic procedures and overcome one of the limitations of robotic surgery. More focused training and earlier exposure to CT surgery through the integrated programs and the 4/3 programs will continue to improve teaching, experience, and performance of CT residents. These programs will integrate all of the aspects of CT training, simulation, robotics, and computer-based knowledge to the benefit of our residents. Some have emphasized the apprentice model, a return to the origins of Halsted training. There certainly is some benefit to the concept. It certainly benefits the attending surgeon to have a resident or assistant who is well versed in their methods. It does allow the resident to identify individual surgeon's preferences. With extended periods of exposure to a single surgeon the two can work more closely together and improve around those procedures done by that attending surgeon. For it to be broadly applied and successful, residents must be exposed to many if not all of the surgeons of a specialty to understand the various techniques, approaches, prejudices, preferences, and special procedures that are done. Limiting the resident's exposure to only a small number of the attending surgeons creates a very narrow experience. The apprentice model may not be appropriate for thoracic track residents who spend a limited amount of time on cardiac surgery, usually 12 months or less. To expose them only to a few surgeons narrows their exposure to cardiac surgery. These concepts will and hopefully improve overtime.

SUMMARY

Patient safety is of utmost importance and always must be part of every conversation about operative teaching. Training must be done in a safe fashion to not expose the patient to undue risk. CT surgery is undergoing an enormous evolution. Tremendous technologic advances occur on an exponential basis. The technological advances seem to evolve every 5 years. One of the great challenges of operative education is how to manage these technological advances and continue to train residents. There is an explosion of knowledge as well as an explosion of technology. Residents must be passionate and dedicated to the acquisition of knowledge and surgical expertise. At present, up to 40% of our residents seek additional training beyond the regular training programs.[21] It is unclear whether this indicates the need for more experience or for specific specialized training. It is probably a combination of both. It does underscore the importance of preparing residents to practice independently in a safe fashion in CT surgery. Although the challenges are many, the dedication of those educators and the willingness to learn on the part of the resident will secure the profession's future. CT surgery is a highly technical, demanding specialty that requires great skill on the part of the surgeons who practice this specialty. There must always be surgeon educators dedicated to training the next generation of surgeons to ensure the highest quality of CT care for patients who require these services. The great surgeon possesses great technical skill and judgment, understands the conduct of an operation, has the flexibility and judgment to change course, and avoids and manages unexpected events. Great surgeons are imbued with "GRIT"!

REFERENCES

1. Vinden C, Malthaner R, McGee J, et al. Teaching surgery takes time: the impact of surgical education on time in the operating room. Can J Surg 2016; 59(2):87–92.
2. Advani V, Ahad S, Gonczy C, et al. Does resident involvement effect surgical times and complication rates during laparoscopic appendectomy for uncomplicated appendicitis? An analysis of 16,849 cases from the ACS-NSQIP. Am J Surg 2012;203:347–52.
3. Philibert I, Friedmann P, Williams WT. New requirements for resident duty hours. JAMA 2002;299: 1112–4.
4. Papandria D, Rhee D, Ortega G, et al. Assessing trainee impact on operative time for common general surgical procedures in ACS-NSQIP. J Surg Educ 2012;69:149–55.
5. Jiang R, Liu Y, Ward KC, et al. Excess cost and predictive factors of esophagectomy complications in the SEER-Medicare database. Ann Thorac Surg 2018;106(5):1484–91.
6. Geller AD, Zheng H, Auchincloss H, et al. Relative incremental cost of postoperative complications of esophagectomy. Semin Thorac Cardiovasc Surg 2018;31(2):290–9.
7. Patel SP, Gauger PG, Brown DL, et al. Resident participation does not affect surgical outcomes, despite introduction of new techniques. J Am Coll Surg 2010;211:540.
8. Bloom JP, Heng EE, Auchincloss HG, et al. Cardiac surgery trainees as "skin-to-skin" operating surgeons: midterm outcomes. Presented at Southern Thoracic Surgical Association 65th Annual Meeting. Amelia Island, November 8, 2018.
9. Lewis FR, Klingensmith ME. Issues in general surgery residency training. Ann Surg 2012;256:553–9.
10. Connors RC, Doty JR, Bull DA, et al. Effect of work-hour restriction on operative experience in cardiothoracic surgical residency training. J Thorac Cardiovasc Surg 2009;137:710–3.
11. Wojcik BM, Fong ZV, Patel MS, et al. Structured operative autonomy: an institutional approach to enhancing surgical resident education without impacting patient outcomes. J Am Coll Surg 2017; 225(6):713–24.
12. Ericsson KA. Acquisition and maintenance of medical expertise: a perspective from the expert-performance approach with deliberate practice. Acad Med 2015;90:1471–86.
13. Ericsson KA, Pool R. Peak: secrets from the new science of expertise. New York: Houghton Mifflan Harcourt; 2016.
14. Roberts NK, Williams RG, Kim MJ, et al. The briefing, intraoperative teaching, debriefing model for teaching in the operating room. J Am Coll Surg 2009;208:299–303.
15. DaRosa DA, Zwishenberger JB, Meyerson SL, et al. A theory-based model for teaching and assessing residents in the operating room. J Surg Educ 2013; 70:24–30.

16. Bohnen JD, George BC, Williams RG, et al. The feasibility of real-time intraoperative performance assessment with SIMPL (System for Improving and Measuring Procedural Learning): early experience from a multi-institutional trial. J Surg Educ 2016; 73(6):e118–30.

17. Morse CR. Minimally invasive Ivor Lewis esophagectomy: how I teach it. Ann Thorac Surg 2018;106: 1283–7.

18. Lombardi V. The Essential Vince Lombardi: words and wisdom to motivate, inspire and win. New York: McGraw Hill; 2003. p. 135.

19. Ten Cate O, Hart D, Ankel F, et al. International competency-based medical education collaborators. Entrustment decision making in clinical training. Acad Med 2016; 91(2):191–8.

20. Duckworth A. Grit: the power of passion and perseverance. New York: Scribner, Simon and Schuster; 2016.

21. Tchantchaleishvili V, LaPar DJ, Stephens EH, et al. Current integrated cardiothoracic surgery residents: a Thoracic Surgery Residents Association survey. Ann Thorac Surg 2015;99(3):1040–7.

Flipping the Classroom
How to Optimize Learning in the Didactic Setting

Joshua L. Hermsen, MD[a],*, Nahush A. Mokadam, MD[b],
Edward D. Verrier, MD[c]

KEYWORDS

- Flipping the classroom • Surgery resident education • Multimedia learning • Death by power point

KEY POINTS

- Effective didactic classroom learning is still an essential component of surgical education.
- Flipping the classroom is an attempt for didactic education to be more learner-centric than teacher-centric.
- Case-based learning opportunities are often most effective.
- "Lecture" retention is low as a learning modality but can be enhanced with multimedia presentation.
- Power Point multimedia presentations can be a double-edged sword when not used properly.

INTRODUCTION

In a surgical residency there are many settings for learning, but classrooms and lecture halls remain important venues for interaction between educators and learners. The goal is deep, rather than superficial, learning, and that means the goal of a learning interaction is to get knowledge into the long-term rather than short-term memory of the learner. Some facts are known about learning in the didactic setting:

1. The setting and format of lectures have an impact on learner retention.[1,2]
2. The attention span of most adult learners is approximately 10 minutes[2] (**Fig. 1**) and most learners have a steep "forgetting curve" unless information is repeated several times[3] (**Fig. 2**).
3. In contrast to other learning opportunities, lectures are probably the least effective methodology leading to long-term memory retention[4] (**Fig. 3**).
4. Different learners may have a preferred neural pathway of learning[5] (visual/auditory).
5. Adults learn differently than children.[6]
6. Neural plasticity remains active throughout life, so even older learners can learn new things.[7]

Clearly, the desired goal of any interaction between teacher and student is for the student to learn and retain something new they did not know previously or increase the breadth and depth of knowledge in areas already available within the working memory. This is a challenging and complex task for which there are numerous educational (both learning and instructional) theories available that shed light on the optimal methodology to achieve "deep" and sustained learning.[8] In surgery, there are numerous physical spaces where learning occurs that include the operating

Disclosure: The authors have nothing to disclose.
[a] University of Wisconsin Hospital and Clinics, 600 Highland Avenue, Clinical Sciences Center, H4/352, Madison, WI 53792-7375, USA; [b] Division of Cardiac Surgery, Ohio State University, N-825 Doan Hall, 410 West 10th Avenue, Columbus, OH 43210, USA; [c] Division of Cardiothoracic Surgery, Department of Surgery, University of Washington, 1959 NE Pacific Street, Seattle WA 98195, USA
* Corresponding author.
E-mail address: jlhermsen@wisc.edu

Thorac Surg Clin 29 (2019) 279–284
https://doi.org/10.1016/j.thorsurg.2019.04.002
1547-4127/19/© 2019 Elsevier Inc. All rights reserved.

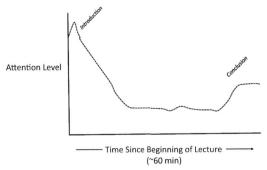

Fig. 1. Learner attention span in lecture presentations: note the rise in attention at the end when the presenter notes: "In conclusion....". (*Adapted from* http://www.scientificleaders.com/presentations; with permission.)

room, the patient's bedside, in the hallways, at home, at meetings, or in the classroom. This article focuses on the classic didactic settings of the classroom and lecture hall and hopefully compliments the other articles in this symposium on adult educational theory, optimizing education in the operating room, e-learning, and self-learning.

Some learning principles apply to all learning environments. The focus of this article is broadly applicable to more than simply surgical education in the classroom because many of the older theories of learning (pedagogy, Socratic methods) are being challenged not only in medical or surgical education but also at introductory levels of learning such as kindergarten, and all the way through university.[9]

Pedagogy classically has been the study of how knowledge and skills are exchanged in an educational context and it considers the interactions that

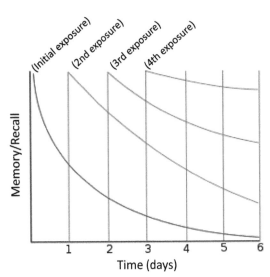

Fig. 2. Ebbinghaus forgetting curve: repetition is essential to long-term retention of knowledge.

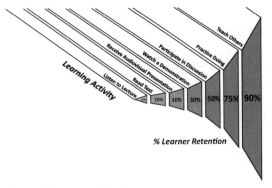

Fig. 3. The cone of learning.

take place during learning.[6] Pedagogy is often thought of as the act of teaching and therefore this type of education is "teacher-centric" or top-down rather than "learner-centric" or bottom-up. Pedagogy has been the dominant learning theory for centuries, and used in almost every classroom setting. In Pedagogy, "I, as the teacher, have all this knowledge or experience and will teach you everything I think you need to know on a particular topic over a specified time frame." The student is viewed as an absorbent sponge. The paradox of Pedagogy is that it requires the learner to be attentive to, and focused on, the content, while at the same time simply remaining a passive recipient of knowledge.

In contrast, andragogy has recently emerged as a more useful learning theory for adults. It is based on the premise, developed by Malcolm Knowles, that adults bring an existing foundation of knowledge and experience to any learning opportunity, are self-directed, and do best when the learning interaction is experiential.[6] Adult learners also approach new learning with an established learning style that may prejudice their acceptance of lecture-based instruction. Experiential learning theory is based on the following concepts: learning is a process that requires engagement and feedback; all learning is *relearning*; learning requires resolution of conceptual conflict; learning involves integrative functioning; learning results from synergy between the learner and the environment; learning is the process of creating knowledge.[10] The concepts of experiential learning theory are integral in adult learning theory—active involvement in goals, building on previous knowledge, intrinsic motivation, and responsibility.[11]

Therefore, in andragogy the role of educators and teachers is redefined to being that learning facilitators.[3] In the andragogic model, "My goal as an educator is not to teach you all I know but rather fill in the gaps related to what you do not yet know or understand." The corollary concept is that learners can maximize learning, by preparing for the lecture and leading the discussion in the class-room. The learner's gaps in knowledge will be readily evident to the teacher who can work to fill such gaps. The methodology used by the educator to fill these gaps (eg, Socratic, peda-gogy) becomes much less important when used for this purpose given its presentation to the learner at a specific point in a situation rich with context. This "flipped classroom" represents a much higher level of learning with greater retention as opposed to simply listening (see **Fig. 3**).

LECTURING AND PUBLIC SPEAKING

Many thoracic surgeons are called on to communi-cate and teach more formally in arenas such as classrooms, lecture halls, visiting professorships, or national meetings. Many surgeons simply as-sume that because they are master surgeons, they are also gifted lecturers or educators.[12] There is both an art and science to preparing and deliv-ering a message that will be processed and remembered by the learner.[13]

The first concept is the preparation of the mes-sage and recognizing the intended audience. To be effective one cannot simply pull off the shelf an out of date, stale, Power Point lecture. There are many books written about effective presenta-tions, but the most recent insights into speaking or lecturing have come from the success of the popular TED series lectures. Carmen Gallo in his book "Talk like Ted: The 9 speaking secrets of the world's top mind" writes about: unleashing the master within, mastering the art of storytelling, have a conversation, teach me something new, deliver jaw dropping moments, lighten up, stick to the 18-minute rule, paint a mental picture with a multisensory experience, and stay in your lane.[13] Not every medical lecture has to resonate like a TED talk but the principles of communication are important and often overlooked in surgical presentations.[14] Almost all modern educators

understand the basic importance of multimedia in preparing and delivering a talk as almost all lec-tures are now based on a slide deck, usually in the Power Point format. However, simply creating dig-ital slides does not necessarily satisfy many of the important TED tenets.

A leading cognitive theory of multimedia learning developed and promoted by Richard Mayer,[5] is based on 3 main assumptions: there are 2 separate channels (auditory and visual) for processing information (dual-coding theory); there is limited channel capacity (cognitive load with either visual or auditory signals), and that learning is an active process of filtering, selecting, orga-nizing, and integrating information based on previ-ous knowledge (**Fig. 4**). There are many implications of these theories for learning in cardiothoracic surgical education because so much of how we approach didactic learning is based on multimedia presentations. Simplified from the original 12 principles of multimedia learning[5] we should understand that:

- People learn better when extraneous words, pictures, and sounds are excluded rather than included.
- People learn better from graphics and narra-tion than from graphics, narration, and text (conflicting cognitive overload).
- People learn better from words and pictures than from words alone.
- People learn better when corresponding words and pictures are presented near rather than far from each other on the page or screen and when presented simultaneously rather than successively.
- The quality and style of auditory presentation is essential for audience engagement.
- People learn better when they are building on a foundation rather than creating one.
- People learn better from multimedia lessons when words are in conversational style rather than formal style.

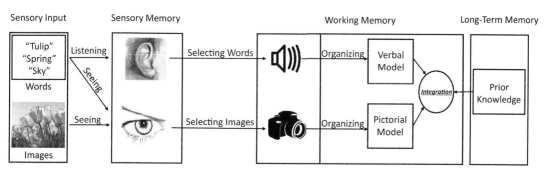

Fig. 4. Mayer multimedia theory of learning: (1) dual coding theory (auditory and visual), (2) there is limited channel capacity (cognitive load), and (3) learning is an active process.

In this multimedia cognitive theory, there is a different role for the 3 memory stores: sensory (which receives stimuli and stores it for a very short time), working (where we actively process information to create mental constructs), and long-term (the repository of all things learned). Multimedia learning presents the idea that the brain does not interpret a multimedia presentation in a mutually exclusive fashion, rather, these elements are selected and organized dynamically to produce logical useable mental constructs with the goal of getting information into retrievable, long-term memory.[15]

Avoid death by Power Point (**Box 1**): when Power Point is used as a crutch for quality in any presentation, rather than a supplementary tool, learning easily gets lost. In any presentation, the media is not the message; the speaker is the expert and they must deliver the message by engaging the audience and retaining their attention. If the teacher does not understand their role as educator, an expert and prepared communicator, the message will get lost in huge data slides, multiple bullet points with unclear emphasis, and uninterpretable messages.

FLIPPING THE CLASSROOM

Flipping the classroom is not a new concept in learning but has recently obtained more notice with the availability of new e-learning tools, learning management systems, and the foundational work in children popularized by Sal Khan in his work: "The One World Schoolhouse: Education Reimagined."[16] In the flipped classroom model, the traditional lecture or reading assignment is included in the learner's curriculum and assigned as homework or preparatory reading for the classroom interaction.[17] In cardiothoracic surgery resident education we have created a progressive curriculum[18] that leverages a learning management system (Learn CT Surgery), a content system (The Brain), and soon (in press) 3 digital textbooks (STS Textbook and Cardiothoracic Surgery) covering all aspects of thoracic, adult cardiac, and congenital heart surgery. Importantly all of these resources are housed within, and managed by, the Society of Thoracic Surgery.

In the flipped classroom model, in-class time is redefined and spent on collaborative, inquiry-based, often case-based active learning. Student-centered instructional models, including the flipped classroom, are grounded in the constructivist theory of learning, whereby learners construct knowledge for themselves. Each learner actively constructs meaning (learns) as new information is linked to previous knowledge and experience.[19] The principles (**Box 2**) are all consistent

---

Box 1
Multimedia presentations: avoiding "death by power point"

- Understand the principles of multimedia learning
- Remember this is about YOU and the MESSAGE
- Engage your audience, make eye contact
- Keep the slides simple (KISS principle)
- Three key elements to slide: arrangement, visual elements, movement
- Avoid bullet points
- Distinguish between presentation and a document
- Avoid big data slides with little red boxes
- Don't turn your back on the audience
- Don't read off the slides
- Make sure videos work
- Rehearse/warm up: reduce, record, repeat
- For longer presentations, tell a story
- Favor images over text (easier to remember)

Box 2
Principles for "flipping the classroom"

- Define clear learning objectives of didactic session
- Limit focus; avoid unrealistic "contentomegally"
- Understand principles of adult learning
- Case-based discussions usually work best
- Avoid long 60-minute, out of date, top-down lectures
- Understand principles of multimedia presentations
- Learner preparation is important/essential
- Effective educator preparation usually requires instruction
- Include assessment tools when possible
- Tailor message/design to different needs of learners (student, resident, faculty)
- Allow adequate time for educator and learner preparation
- Learn how to include e-learning resources as adjuncts to didactic sessions (content management, learning management, knowledge management systems, curriculum)
- Recognize senior faculty often like to hear themselves talk

with currently popular theories of adult learning. The core principle of constructivism applied to learning is that the environment is learner-centered and learning is an active rather than passive endeavor. Such an approach to surgical learning emphasizes self-direction, active inquiry, independence, and individuality. The instructor's role is to foster critical reflection and facilitate the application and deeper understanding of new concepts.[20] *This concept becomes extremely important in light of work duty hour restrictions for time available in the hospital, and the clear need for medical students and residents to use their learning time out of the hospital productively.* The reported use of flipped classrooms, based on published articles, in graduate medical education has significantly increased in the past several years.[21] Current research evidence also shows that the flipped classroom has many potential advantages:

- Increased opportunities to provide individualized education to learners and to incorporate evidence-based teaching techniques into existing interactions. As surgical educators this is important as we often have the need to teach at multiple levels during the same didactic session as teaching conference attendees may include senior residents, junior residents, medical students, perfusionists, nurse practitioners, physician assistants, and colleagues in medicine or anesthesiology.
- Once past the initial investment phase in educational culture change, the approach may allow educators to optimize their time or share their time with other peer surgical colleagues without having to prepare multiple lectures.
- Flipped classrooms, if constructed correctly, may increase educator-student interaction time as the educator is present when students attempt to analyze and apply new knowledge.
- Active learning techniques—such as teamwork, debates, and case studies—prompt student engagement and encourage them to explore attitudes and values while fostering student-centered learning and motivation to acquire new knowledge; all important traits beyond medical knowledge.[22]
- Maybe most importantly, active learning also stimulates the higher-order thinking, problem solving, critical analysis and decision making skills crucial for surgeons.

There are many factors that can contribute to successful implementation of a flipped classroom. Probably the most important is faculty buy-in. Past generations of learners in medicine were taught in the classroom in the teacher-centric approach with huge slide show-type presentations and minimal teacher-learner interaction. That may have worked for a certain generation of learners when the body of knowledge was less, index cases were simpler (coronary artery bypass grafts, aortic valves, lobectomies) and more plentiful, and work hours were more liberal. The flipped method represents a significant shift away from traditional 1-hour Power Point-based lectures, and there is an initial faculty effort required to create and organize online materials for learners to review before holding interactive in-class sessions. One payoff for this effort is the relative ease of creating assessment tools to enhance overall educational accountability within the flipped classroom model. The good news is that many of the digital and online educational content resources have already been created in cardiothoracic surgery through the JCTSE, STS, AATS, EJCTS, TSDA, and CTS. Net. In addition, a state of the art, digital textbook is being created by the STS and should be available globally by fall 2019. Excellent introductory articles on flipping the classroom have been written by Jennifer Moffett in 2015[23] and Catherine Lewis for the Bulletin of the American College of Surgeons in 2016.[17]

SUMMARY

In this article we have tried to emphasize the art and science of effective classroom teaching. The surgical educator must understand that "flipping the classroom" and preparing effective presentations takes time and effort. This represents a fundamental change in the role of surgeon as educator and requires practice and an arduous change of educational culture and mindset.[20,24] When done well the master surgeon has the opportunity to extend their positive influence well beyond the operating room.

REFERENCES

1. Gilke RM, Johnson MR, Knight KE, et al. Recall of lecture information: a question of what, when, and where. Med Educ 1982;16(5):264–8.
2. Prober CG, Heath C. Lecture halls without lectures—a proposal for medical education. N Engl J Med 2012;366(18):1657–9.
3. Schacter DL. The seven sins of memory: how the mind forgets and remembers. Boston: Houghton Mifflin; 2001. ISBN 978-0-618-21919-3.
4. Kolb AY, Kolb DA. Learning styles and learning spaces: enhancing experiential learning in higher education. Acad Manag Learn Educ 2005;4:193–212.

5. Mayer RE. Multimedia learning. Cambridge (United Kingdom): Cambridge University Press; 2012.

6. Knowles MS. The modern practice of adult education. New York: Adult Education Company; 1980.

7. Debarnot U, Sperduti M, Di Rienzo F, et al. Expert bodies, expert minds: how physical and mental training shape the brain. Front Hum Neurosci 2014;8:1–15.

8. Taylor DCM, Hamdy H. Adult learning theories: implications for learning and teaching in medical education: AMME guide No. 83. Med Teach 2013; 35(11):E1561–72.

9. Robinson K. Out of our minds: learning to be creative. West Sussex (United Kingdom): Capstone; 2011.

10. Kolb DA. Experiential learning: experience as the source of learning and development. Englewood Cliffs (New Jersey): Prentice Hall; 1984.

11. Goldman S. The educational Kanban: promoting effective self-directed adult learning in medical education. Acad Med 2009;84:927–34.

12. Verrier ED. The elite athlete...the master surgeon. J Am Coll Surg 2016;224(3):225–35.

13. Gallo C. Talk like Ted: the 9 public speaking secrets of the world's top minds. New York: St Martin's Press; 2014.

14. Vaporciyan AA, Yang SC, Baker CJ, et al. Cardiothoracic surgery residency training: past, present and future. J Thorac Cardiovasc Surg 2013;146:759–67.

15. Duarte N. Slideology: the art and science of creating great presentations. Sebastopol (CA): O'Reilly Media; 2008.

16. Khan S. The one world schoolhouse: education reimagined. London: Hodder & Stoughton; 2012.

17. Lewis CE. The flipped classroom: abandon the sage on the stage, and embrace the guide on the side. Bulle Am Coll Surg. Available at: https://www.facs.org/education/division-of-education/publications/rise/articles/flipped.

18. Duarte N. Resonate: present visual stories that transform audiences. Hoboken (NJ): John Wiley & Sons; 2010.

19. Oustaee R, Abd. Kadir S, Asimiran S. A review of constructivist teaching practices. Middle East J Sci 2014;19:145–52.

20. Mokadam NA, Dardas TF, Hermsen J, et al. Flipping the classroom: case-based learning, accountability, assessment, and feedback leads to a favorable change in culture. J Thorac Cardiovasc Surg 2016; 153(4):987–96.e1.

21. King AM, Gottlieb M, Mitzman J, et al. Flipping the classroom in graduate medical education: a systematic review. J Grad Med Educ 2019;11(1):18–29.

22. McLaughlin JE, Roth MT, Glatt DM, et al. The flipped classroom: a course redesign to foster learning and engagement in a health professions school. Acad Med 2014;89(2):236–43.

23. Moffett J. Twelve tips for "flipping" the classroom. Med Teach 2015;37(4):331–6.

24. Heath C, Heath D. Switch: how to change things when change is hard. New York: Broadway Books; 2010.

E-Learning Trends and How to Apply Them to Thoracic Surgery Education

Lauren Aloia, BA[a], Ara A. Vaporciyan, MD, MHPE[b],*

KEYWORDS

- E-learning • Formative assessment • Internet • Thoracic surgery • Web-based learning
- Online learning • Internet-based learning • Computer-assisted instruction

KEY POINTS

- The current system of graduate medical education, an apprenticeship model, is successful but labor intensive and its effective use is threatened by external changes.
- E-learning systems, coupled with built-in formative assessments, have demonstrated the ability to teach basic concepts through independent learning.
- These systems are already in place in cardiothoracic surgical education in North America.
- Application of E-learning allows instructors to selectively apply apprenticeship when teaching more complex concepts, concepts that are harder to teach in an E-learning environment.

INTRODUCTION

Education in all fields is vastly different today than it was 20 years ago. Today, the Internet is a powerful tool that students and educators use to supplement or replace traditional learning. This technique is referred to as E-learning, or the use of Internet technologies, to deliver a broad array of solutions that enhance knowledge and performance.[1] E-learning is also called Web-based learning, online learning, internet-based learning, and computer-assisted instruction among many others.[1]

Medical education has many long established approaches to learning using face-to-face teacher-centered models.[2] As medicine has evolved the focus on medical education has drifted. Kenneth Ludmere outlines the series of changes from the publication of the Flexner Report in 1910 to the rise of managed care in the 2000s. After Flexner's report led to the closure of nearly two-thirds of the medical schools, the remaining academic medical centers focused almost exclusively on medical education. In the 50s and 60s,

the recognition of the value of medical research with an associated increase in funding led to an increasing focus on research. In the 90s, when funding for research declined and a focus on patient outcomes increased academic centers turned to increased clinical productivity as their primary focus, research remained number 2 and attention on education declined.

But it is not just the changing focus of academic centers that dilutes education. Medical education has always mirrored an apprenticeship. It heavily depends on one-on-one teaching, mostly at the bedside or in the operating room, by a cadre of dedicated clinical instructors. It is highly effective but requires a significant time commitment. Unfortunately, even the most dedicated clinical teacher is challenged due to several external forces. The obvious first is a competition for time. Increasing documentation requirements, the need to be more productive both clinically and academically, as well as a host of other factors decrease the time a clinician can devote to teaching. Second is an increasing complexity of cases. Changes in

Disclosure Statement: The authors have nothing to disclose.
[a] Lauren Aloia 6035 Francis Street, Jupiter, FL 33458, USA; [b] Department of Thoracic and Cardiovascular Surgery, 1515 Holcombe Boulevard, Box 1489, Houston, TX 77030, USA
* Corresponding author.
E-mail address: avaporci@mdanderson.org

1547-4127/19/© 2019 Elsevier Inc. All rights reserved.

thoracic.theclinics.com

medical practice, especially in thoracic surgery, have decreased the volume of simple cases, which are now addressed with nonsurgical approaches. The result is an inability to gradually move a trainee through a series of easier cases before tackling the more challenging ones. Third is an increasing scrutiny on outcomes. Of course, this is not a bad thing; we all want to raise the quality of our profession. However, when coupled with increasing case complexity, this makes the challenges of educating a novice learner even greater. Finally, there is the exponential growth in medical knowledge, consider it Moore's law as applied to medicine. Examine the increase in publications focused on cardiothoracic surgery (**Fig. 1**). During a 2-year fellowship in 2015, a trainee experienced nearly 10,000 new publications relevant to his or her field of study. Compare that trainee with the same trainee in 1970 who saw less than 2000 publications. How can a trainee possibly filter through all this information? Of all these issues faced as educators, this is perhaps the most insidious and unrelenting. The ability to keep up with the advance of knowledge will continually become more and more challenging.

In this article, the authors' aim is not to diminish the age-old apprenticeship model of education in cardiothoracic surgery. Some complex medical decision making and certainly technical skills can only be taught face-to-face. Knowledge, especially what the trainees must acquire, comes in a hierarchy of levels (**Fig. 2**).[3] Adapting and integrating E-learning elements into traditional methods could be the solution that results in high levels of learner satisfaction.[4] By focusing E-learning on lower level knowledge, such as remembering and understanding, we can free up time for faculty to teach the harder skills that are best learned through face-to-face interactions.

The authors examine a few popular trends in E-learning and how to integrate them into thoracic surgery education programs: learning management systems and content curation and formative assessments.

LEARNING MANAGEMENT SYSTEMS AND CONTENT CURATION

A learning management system (LMS) is a Web-based software application that allows educational organizations or programs to deliver content and resources to their learners.[5] LMSs support a range of uses from delivering online courses, housing content, administering quizzes, and providing reports. With many systems, educators have the option to use the LMS in a way that best supports their needs. An LMS can be viewed as the basis of an E-learning environment.

The key benefits of using an LMS include the ability to centralize learning, create the ability to update material in a timely manner, provide learners the flexibility over timing and pace (self-directed learning), and finally support real-time tracking and reporting. Although an LMS includes content, it is more than simply a content management system (CMS). A CMS simply houses content and makes it available. It is the ability of an LMS to track the progress of the users, that is, the learners, that distinguishes it from a CMS. Still, content is integral to most LMS platforms so how that content is arranged and presented is a key

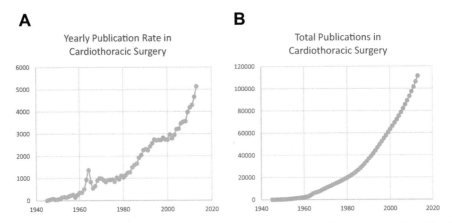

Fig. 1. The exponential increase in publications focused on a subset of cardiothoracic surgical publications from 1945 through 2013. All articles listed in Medline linked to the following MeSH headings were collected: "Thoracic Surgery," "Cardiovascular Surgical Procedures," "Heart Transplantation," "Lung Neoplasm/[Surgery]," "Esophageal Neoplasm/[Surgery]," "Heart Valve Prosthesis," "Heart Valve Prosthesis Implantation." (*A*) The amount of publications produced each year. (*B*) The total articles published to date.

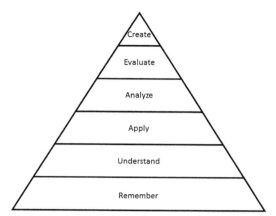

Fig. 2. Adaptation of Bloom's taxonomy of knowledge. (*Adapted from* Anderson LW, Krathwohl DR, Airasian PW, et al. A taxonomy for learning, teaching and assessing. New York: Addison Wesley Longman, Inc; 2001. p. 31; with permission)

feature of those LMSs that include content management.

These platforms are central to all distance learning activities and have become ubiquitous in K-12 and college education. Blackboard is a proprietary LMS platform providing K-12, higher education, government and business education opportunities. University of Phoenix and Southern New Hampshire University are 2 well-recognized examples of higher education applications.

Content curation is the process of organizing and presenting information on the Web in an organized manner, developed around a common theme. Content curators provide a customized, vetted selection of the best, most relevant resources. By combining the use of an LMS and content curation for thoracic surgery education, educators are able to provide their learners with a wealth of on-demand information and eliminate unneeded content. These 2 E-learning tactics can essentially replace Web searching.

In thoracic surgery, the educators have begun to implement these techniques. They initially piloted the concept of an LMS in the fall of 2013.[6] Using an open-source LMS platform (MOODLE: Modular Object-Oriented Dynamic Learning Environment) 4 courses were created that addressed aspects of tracheal disorders, a subject where trainees consistently performed poorly during the ABTS written examination. Each course addressed a subject relevant to diagnosing and treating patients with tracheal disease. They included pulmonary physiology and assessment, radiographic and surgical

anatomy of the trachea, disorders of the trachea and bronchus, and tracheal and bronchial surgery. Each course included reading material relevant to the subject as well as a bank of multiple choice questions. The courses included a quiz that was randomly created for each learner from the available relevant bank of questions. To "pass" a course the trainee would need to obtain a 90% score. They could take the quiz as often as they liked but the quiz was different each time they took it. The course was distributed to 19 trainees in 4 institutions across the United States. The courses were very well received and analysis of the quiz scores demonstrated that the trainees were able to gain knowledge independently demonstrating a proof of concept.

Based on this work, the Joint Council, which had funded the original pilot, was given permission by its board of directors to expand this platform to all thoracic surgical trainees and simultaneously address all relevant topics in cardiothoracic surgery. Initially the authors elected to remain on the MOODLE platform, but limitations of this platform required that they move to a more responsive platform created by Astute Technologies (now owned by Echo360, Inc.). The new platform maintained the ability to present content relevant to the subject being addressed and link each section to a relevant bank of MCQ's that trainees could access for assessments (see later discussion). The new platform also allowed individual programs to have some control of the content they presented their trainees. They could upload content that was visible just to their trainees along with accessing the nationally selected content.

However, what the authors quickly recognized was the need to curate content. Without a single resource to address all topics they were forced to cobble together content to address each of the topics. This included older articles that were open source, some textbooks for which they had to pay significant fees to the publishers, some narrated PowerPoint lectures, and even a few videos. The wide variety of sources meant that without oversight significant overlap of the content would develop. Many articles were more detailed than necessary and some book chapters veered off topic. A structured editorial oversight was needed to ensure that the content was as on point as possible with the least amount of gaps or overlap.

This was a herculean task when coupled with the rapidly expanding content that was alluded to earlier. The authors' solution has been to create their own wiki-style textbook that will be tied directly to the curriculum. This will allow us to align the content with the topics presented in the curriculum and simultaneously reduce the cost through a reduction in administrative oversight and fees paid to the publishers. The wiki format will allow editorially reviewed updates to the chapters to be made in real time as opposed to waiting for new editions of a print-bound textbook, which are usually out of date by the time they are published. The Society of Thoracic Surgeons, after assuming control of the Joint Council, has graciously assisted with the capital costs of creating such a textbook and an anticipated release is in the summer of 2019.

FORMATIVE ASSESSMENT

Formative assessments, increasingly being referred to as just assessments, is "the process used by teachers and students to recognize and respond to student learning in order to enhance that learning, during the learning."[7] The primary purpose of these assessments is to illuminate learner knowledge gaps by providing feedback during the teaching process. However, formative assessment feedback is difficult for clinical faculty to provide due to the increasing time constraints and other external pressures. Applying formative assessments into E-learning environments automates feedback and eliminates the need for faculty to be present; this also gives students the ability to actively assess themselves.[8]

In a 2004 study, Dr Tzu-Hua Wang developed the Formative Assessment Module of the Web-based Assessment and Test Analysis System (FAM-WATA). FAM-WATA helps educators construct an assessment-centered E-learning environment through multiple-choice formative assessments.[7] Wang's study was composed of 6 main strategies, all of which proved to achieve better learning effectiveness (**Box 1**).

Box 1 FAM-WATA strategies
1. Repeat the test
2. Answers are not given
3. Ask questions
4. Monitoring answering history
5. Query scores
6. All pass and then reward.

Briefly, FAM-WATA provides learners with random multiple-choice questions from the database with random arrangement of the answer options. When a learner answers a question correctly 3 times consecutively, FAM-WATA is confident enough that the learner understands the concept and removes the question from the test. Eventually, all questions will be removed and the learner will "pass the test."[8] This concept supports strategies 1 and 2. FAM-WATA supports the third strategy, "ask questions," by directing learners to reference materials that will help them answer the questions they answered incorrectly. Making sure the feedback is timely is a vital aspect of this strategy. A large advantage of using assessments in conjunction with E-learning is that learners can monitor their own learning and progress. Once users pass the test, FAM-WATA provides them with their own answering history as well as the answering history of others. This supports strategy number 4. Similar to strategy number 4, strategy number 5, "query scores", allows learners to look up the scores and progress of their peers. This is to stimulate and encourage competition among the group. Finally, FAM-WATA congratulates learners on passing the test as a way to encourage learners and generate a sense of achievement.

The power of self-testing as a learning strategy was demonstrated in multiple other studies.[9,10] In one example, subjects were given an opportunity to study a text passage either for two 7-minute periods or for 1 period and test their recall for the subsequent 7 minutes. The group that mixed study with testing had much better recall 2 days and 1 week later than the group that simply engaged in study. Later work demonstrated that testing continued to enhance retention when it occupied up to 75% of the time allocated to studying and self-testing.

A well-known example of real-life application of this approach is seen in Kahn Academy. Their approach include a rich library of content embedded within their LMS, but integral to their environment is self-directed testing that incorporates all the elements of FAM-WATA. Students can take tests repeatedly. They earn badges as they successfully complete each section. Gaps in a student' knowledge, exposed during testing, are addressed by referring the student directly to the relevant Kahn video.

In thoracic surgery the authors have also begun to implement these techniques. Not all knowledge can be assessed easily. Knowledge comes in many forms and the more complex the concept the more the assessment required. **Fig. 2** is an example of one of the taxonomies of the types of knowledge. Lower levels of knowledge such as remembering, understanding, and applying include processes such as recognizing, interpreting, classifying, inferring, and executing. If one considers thoracic surgery, some examples of these forms of knowledge include recognition of anatomic structures, interpreting findings on a radiograph, classifying patients according to stage, inferring a diagnosis based on test results, and executing the calculation of postoperative predicted pulmonary function. Higher level of knowledge, evaluating and creating, includes processes such as checking, generating, and producing. Examples might include checking the adequacy of a bronchial closure or an anatomic dissection, generating a treatment plan, and producing a new approach when faced with an intraoperative dilemma.

It becomes clear that the easier the knowledge type, the easier the type of testing needed to assess it. Most remembering and understanding (and even some applying) can be assessed through well-constructed multiple-choice questions. For the more advanced knowledge types, more complex testing is required. Long answer formats, written responses, or, most commonly, oral formats are used to assess these more complex forms of knowledge. These latter testing formats are difficult to implement in a self-directed E-learning environment. However, multiple-choice questions can be administered, graded, and linked to specific content all in an automated fashion.

This is exactly what has been done in the E-learning platform currently in production. Although all the elements of the FAM-WATA have not been incorporated yet, many of the key strategies are in place. The tests are constructed randomly by drawing questions from an established question bank. The answers are also randomized. Answers are not given immediately but only after completion of a test. A trainee's quiz history is maintained and each trainee can compare their scores across all trainees nationally. The only gap in the current approach is the "ask question" strategy. Without a uniform and stable content library the authors do not provide suggested readings when a question is answered incorrectly. However, with the development of the new wiki textbooks these 2 may become a possibility. Textbook sections could be linked to each item in the question bank and when answered incorrectly that section of the textbook could be presented to the learner to guide their learning and help close that gap in their knowledge.

SUMMARY

E-learning is an area of astonishing growth. As alluded to by Clayton Christenson it promises to be, and in some sectors already is, a disruptive technology in education.[11] Considering the rate of knowledge growth in medicine compared with K-12 education as well as the other external threats, such as time and increasing case complexity, the value of E-learning approaches in graduate medical education is significant. Simply continuing with the same approaches is doomed to failure. Similarly, the application of the new understanding of how people learn is made possible with the application of E-learning technology. The ability to allow real-time self-testing strategies must be incorporated. Although the authors' prior reliance on faculty-led assessments was effective, the rate of knowledge growth and the demands placed on their clinical faculty only make it untenable as a sole solution. Combining these 2 modalities into the educational environment is an imperative. It is also what the new learners will demand, as they will be entering the learning environment having come from one that is rich in these approaches. To not embrace them and implement them will erode their interest in our field.

This article only identifies 2 of the many areas of E-learning. The authors focus on those that they have been able to incorporate to date. It is hoped that other approaches will make their way into the educational environment and continue to enhance the educational system for cardiothoracic surgical training.

REFERENCES

1. Ruiz JG, Mintzer MJ, Leipzig RM. The impact of E-Learning in medical education. Acad Med 2006; 81:207–12.
2. O'Doherty D, Dromey M, Lougheed J, et al. Barriers and solutions to online learning in medical education – An Integrative Review. BMC Med Educ 2018;18: 130.
3. Anderson LW, Krathwohl DR, Airasian PW, et al. A taxonomy for learning, teaching and assessing. New York: Addison Wesley Longman, Inc; 2001.
4. Evgeniou E, Loizou P. The theoretical base of E-learning and its role in surgical education. J Surg Educ 2012;69(5):665–9.
5. Muthalan N. LMS trends and how they impact key players in the ecosystem. eLearning Industry. Available at: https://elearningindustry.com/lms-trends-impact-key-players-ecosystem. Accessed April 22, 2019.

6. Antonoff MB, Verrier ED, Yang SC, et al. Online learning in thoracic surgical training: promising results of multi-institutional pilot study. Ann Thorac Surg 2014;3:1057–63.

7. Bell B, Cowie B. The characteristics of formative assessment in science education. Sci Ed 2001;85:536–53.

8. Wang T. What strategies are effective for formative assessment in an e-Learning environment? Semantic Scholar. Available at: https://www.semanticscholar.org/paper/What-strategies-are-effective-for-formative-in-anWang/19d5edaf298442f284fb2125809f43cc03b663b8. Accessed April 22, 2019.

9. Roediger HL III, Karpicke JD. Test enhanced learning: taking memory tests improves long-term retention. Psychol Sci 2006;17:249–55.

10. Larson DP, Butler AC, Roediger HL. Repeated testing improves long-term retention relative to repeated study: a randomized controlled trial. Med Educ 2009;43:1174–81.

11. Christensen CM, Johnson CW, Horn MB. Disrupting class: how disruptive innovation will change the way the world learns. New York: McGraw-Hill; 2008.

The Alternative Surgical Curriculum

Stephen C. Yang, MD

KEYWORDS

• Surgical education • Nontechnical skills • Cognitive skills • Teamwork • Communication • Burnout

KEY POINTS

- Interpersonal and cognitive skills are essential for the development of a surgeon in addition to technical skills.
- Interpersonal skills consist of communication, leadership, teamwork, planning/preparation for surgery, and coping with pressure/stress/fatigue.
- Cognitive skills consist of situation awareness, decision making, and developing adaptive strategies.
- Noncognitive traits are important in order to be sensitive to colleagues and family, and include emotional intelligence, grit/resiliency, and implicit bias.

INTRODUCTION

Surgeons have to be human too. Since residency-based surgical training was started in 1889 by Dr. William Halsted at Johns Hopkins Hospital, on-the-job training has largely focused on learning clinical and technical skills. "See one, do one, teach one" are the words that briefly express this traditional method of training. Since then, all surgeons have learned surgery from their seniors in this mechanical way, growing step by step from beginners to experts. Instruction and training on nontechnical skills was lacking.

To prepare residents in training for a successful daily practice, in 1999, the Accreditation Council for Graduate Medical Education (ACGME) developed the 6 core competencies that defined foundational skills that practicing physicians should possess. Educational programs that reflect skills and attributes relevant to patient care were developed but mainly focused on knowledge, patient care, and skills development.

The operating room (OR) is a highly complex and stressful environment that requires interaction between a large interdisciplinary team to achieve successful outcomes for the patient. This requires not only effective procedure-specific technical skills but also a range of nontechnical skills. The importance of these skills is often overlooked and unfortunately can be the source of surgical error. These "softer" skills have been ignored in the past and believed to be a natural skillset, but over time, as a result of several external and generational changes, they have become key components that defines a surgeon's ability.

Many of these topics in this "alternative surgical curriculum" have been covered elsewhere in this monograph. This article focuses on nontechnical skills; some may have successful strategies in curriculum, assessment, and research; others are still in their infancy of validation in a surgeon's armamentarium. This is a brief review on selected topics. Individually, they are stand-alone subjects in published articles and books but believed to be helpful for all cardiothoracic surgeons to be aware of and may be stimulated to read about. Clearly none of these topics are discussed in any depth during residency.

A taxonomy for these skills has been proposed (**Table 1**), breaking down these important

Disclosure Statement: The author has nothing to disclose.
Division of Thoracic Surgery, The Johns Hopkins Medical Institutions, 600 North Wolfe Street, Blalock 240, Baltimore, MD 21287, USA
E-mail address: syang@jhmi.edu
; @SteveYangMD (S.C.Y.)

Thorac Surg Clin 29 (2019) 291–301
https://doi.org/10.1016/j.thorsurg.2019.04.003
1547-4127/19/© 2019 Elsevier Inc. All rights reserved.

Table 1
Proposed taxonomy for nontechnical skills

Interpersonal Skills	Cognitive Skills	Noncognitive Traits
Communication	Situation awareness	Emotional intelligence
Leadership	Mental readiness	Grit and resiliency
Teamwork	Assessing risks	Implicit bias
Briefing/planning/preparation	Anticipating problems	
Resource management	Decision making	
Seeking advice and feedback	Adaptive strategies and flexibility	
Coping with pressure/stress/fatigue	Workload distribution	
	Situation awareness	
	Mental readiness	
	Assessing risks	
	Anticipating problems	

Adapted from Yule S, Flin R, Paterson-Brown S, et al. Nontechnical skills for surgeons in the operating room: a review of the literature. Surgery 2006;139:140-9; with permission.

topics—teamwork, emotional intelligence, leadership, effective communication, deliberate practice, grit, mindset, presence, character, implicit bias, diversity/harassment—into interpersonal and cognitive skills. A third set of skills, the noncognitive traits, is included in this discussion and may overlap with effective communication, but they are associated with an individual's personality, temperament, and attitudes.

In 1994, Helmreich and Schaefer observed operations in a European teaching hospital using 9 categories of "specific behaviors that can be evaluated in terms of their presence or absence and quality that are essential for safe and efficient function."[1] Using this performance categorization for their observations, they identified several instances when errors occurred that were related to inadequate teamwork, failures in preparation, poor communication, and unsatisfactory workload distribution (**Table 2**).

INTERPERSONAL SKILLS
Communication

In the early 2000s when safety became an important issue regarding medical errors, a retrospective review of 258 closed malpractice claims revealed that system factors contributed to error in 82% of cases and that communication breakdown was the leading cause accounting for 24% of these.[2] Communication failures are the central causes of near misses. Obviously, the team that practices good communication in the OR and handoffs between the different levels of care (eg, OR to recovery, shift to shift), contributes to the high performance and outcomes associated with higher case volumes.

Handoffs have become a central issue, especially with limitations in residency work hours, shift work for advance practitioners, and the complexity

of surgical interventions. A clinical handoff is defined as a "transfer of professional responsibility and accountability for some or all aspects of care for a patient, or groups of patients, to another

Table 2
Errors observed in operating theaters classified by behavior category

Behavior Category	Error
Communications/ decisions	Surgeon's failure to inform anesthesiologist
Preparation/ planning/ vigilance	Failure to anticipate events during complex procedures Failure to monitor other team activities
Workload distribution/ distraction avoidance	Surgeon is distracted from making a decision by problems reported from another operating room
Briefings	Failure to brief own team
Inquiry/assertion/ advocacy	Failure to discuss alternative procedure
Interpersonal relationships/ group climate	Hostility and frustrations owing to poor team coordination
Team self-critique	Failure to debrief operation and learn from situation
Leadership/ followership/ concern for tasks	Failure to establish leadership for operating room team
Conflict resolution	Unresolved conflicts between surgical team and anesthesiologists

Adapted from Helmreich RL, Schaefer HG. Team performance in the operating room. In: Bogner M, editor. Human error in medicine. Hillsdale, NJ: Lawrence Erlbaum Associates; 1994. p. 225-53; with permission.

person or professional group on a temporary or permanent basis."[3] This is probably one of the most important skills that new interns should have. It remains critical for patient safety and continuity of care and is logical for clinical efficiency.

In the classic 2001 Institute of Medicine reports *To Err is Human* and *Crossing the Quality Chiasm,* safer surgical care is achieved through robust exchange of clinical information between clinicians and calls for teamwork in the continuity of care.[4] It has been shown, especially among surgeons, that handoffs can often be inaccurate, rushed, and unstructured, if they take place at all.[5–7] Obviously, this has been an intense area of improvement and standardization in the perioperative period.[7,8]

Leadership

Physicians, irrespective of their level of training or practice, require leadership competencies to become more actively involved in the planning, delivery, and transformation of health care and education. Leadership is now recognized as a fundamental characteristic in the ACGME Core Competency of communication skills, and, along with coordination abilities in the OR, 1 of the 3 markers that distinguishes surgeons to minimize error.[9]

Leadership has many definitions. It can be a process by which one influences others to accomplish an objective and directs the organization in a way to make it more cohesive and coherent. Leaders are always held accountable for the successes and failures of the team. There are many theories on how leadership can differ from "management." It is a trait that is learned, acquired, or matured through coaching and mentorship. Thousands of books have been written, with innumerable electronic platforms available through the Internet to foster leadership qualities. However, development of leadership relies on certain personal attributes such as beliefs, ethics, values, and character that make oneself unique.[10]

The interest at all levels is held in high regard, with nearly all individual institutions, medical associations, and specialty societies holding courses and training sessions dedicated to this topic. A partial list of national organizations offering leadership programs specifically for surgeons is listed in **Table 3**.

Leadership in the OR is expected of all surgeons. Much research has been done to identify specific behavior traits essential to lead a team in the OR. This has led to the development of specific taxonomies: elucidator, tone setter, engagement facilitator, delegator, safe space maker, conductor,

Table 3
National programs in leadership

Sponsoring Association	Title
American College of Surgeons	From Operating Room to Boardroom
American College of Surgeons	Residents as Teachers and Leaders
American College of Surgeons	Surgeons as Leaders
Association for Academic Surgery	Leadership Development Program
Brandeis University	Leadership Program for Health Policy and Management
Harvard Medical School	Surgical Leadership Program

and being human.[11,12] These studies concluded that this taxonomy of OR to guide behavior can be used as a basis for developing an OR guiding strategy to improve residents' intraoperative competency, autonomy, and independence.

Teamwork

Communication is closely tied to teamwork. This is the defined as the skills required for working in a team context to ensure that the team has an acceptable shared picture of the situation and can complete tasks effectively.[13] It is essential that this mental model is shared by all on the team, on what is going on currently, and the planned outcome. Internal barriers to communication include language differences, culture, motivation, expectations, past experience, emotions, and differences in seniority. External barriers consist of noise, low or incomprehensible voice, electrical interference, space/time separation, and lack of visual cues. These barriers are more evident with increasing complexity of operations and the added use of other equipment or technology.

Contribution to good teamwork is easier if the team members know one another. Introductions at the beginning of cases or procedures can help to resolve some of these barriers. Knowing the other team members can reduce interpersonal tension and help all stay calm when a disaster occurs. Understanding everyone's skills can increase patience when problems arise, and most would have patience knowing that problems are likely a result of technical challenges rather than incompetence. The creation of a safe and "well-oiled machine" in the OR encourages people to ask for help inside and outside the OR.

Briefing/Planning/Preparation

Similar to the airline industry, the introduction of checklists, time outs and huddles when a case is about to start undoubtedly has contributed to the safety culture and improved various nontechnical skills, which translate into a better operative procedure. Decision making is facilitated by reviewing the operative plan, possible difficulties, and the projected need for other equipment. As discussed previously, this overlaps and enhances communication, teamwork, and leadership. Although it can be viewed as an imposition, review of these checklists, performing the institutional time out protocols, and having a preoperative conference/intraoperative huddle are fundamental for good leadership by showing a commitment to patient safety and recognizing the important role that each team member plays in the OR.

Coping with Stress, Burnout, and Fatigue

The first report about the topic of burnout in surgery was by Wray in 1983.[14] Hundreds of reports from different specialties and analyzed at different learner levels have been published since then, which consistently show that stress and burnout are reported in approximately 40% of surgeons.[15]

The ability to deal with stress and fatigue are important nontechnical skills. One must first be able to acknowledge its existence, recognize how it will affect operative behavior and cognitive skills, and know how to alleviate it to improve performance. Physician burnout is a term for one of the most serious outcomes from stress that overwhelm doctors—chronic emotional exhaustion associated with general diminished interest that could lead to depression and suicide. Obviously, this adversely affects patient care and surgical safety. In a 2010 systematic review of 22 articles regarding acute stress in surgery, based on real OR and simulated situations, the major stressors were the act of surgery itself—unexpected bleeding, room noise, visitors, and other distractions.[16] Open surgery was found to be less stressful than laparoscopic surgery. More senior surgeons seem to handle stress better than their junior colleagues, which translates into the ability to maintain technical skills during times of tension. In addition, during times of duress, cognitive skills decrease, reducing available working memory affecting decision making, perception, and task management. Thus, when judgment is dependent on what is the best workable decision, people can "freeze" if they lack the experience. The cycle perpetuates as uncertainty breeds anxiety.

Numerous surveys regarding burnout in surgeons have revealed similar patterns. The factors independently associated with emotional exhaustion include work–home conflicts, excessive workload, inadequate administrative time, and inability to care for personal health.[17] Burnout was the single greatest predictor of career dissatisfaction and accounted for more of the variation in satisfaction with career and specialty choice than any other personal or professional factor. Emotional exhaustion was inversely associated with career satisfaction and positively associated with consideration of early retirement. Regarding patterns in specialty surgeons, otolaryngologists had the highest burnout rate, but ironically career satisfaction was higher than in other surgical specialties.[17]

Although institutions and departments now focus on well-being and provide programs on enhancing resiliency, this seems to address only the symptoms of stress and burnout rather than the root cause.[18] Residents spend up to 40% of their time doing clerical duties, and only 12% on direct patient care,[19] and similarly, surgical interns spend most of their day on noneducational tasks rather than learning operative or clinical skills.[20] This same pattern continues after training; practicing physicians spend as much as one-sixth of their time with administrative and clerical work directly related to the imposed use of electronic health records.[21]

The deluge of administrative obligation is not likely to change in the near future, so the best efforts in maintaining resiliency are individual efforts to integrate personal and professional life goals. Strategies that may help enhance wellness should focus on actively nurturing, practicing, and protecting well-being on all levels: physical, psychological, emotional, and spiritual.[17]

Fatigue is a state of sleepiness by feeling drowsy or tired. This results in a reduced ability to maintain concentration, make decisions, and carry out skilled tasks. Lack of sleep is the most common cause of fatigue. This affects thinking and decision making; both become less clear, less imaginative, and less flexible while accepting lower standards of performance. It translates into a major cause of traffic and health care accidents. Reduction of work hours and allowing for quality sleep within 1 to 2 days after sleep deprivation can overcome fatigue and reduce errors.[22] The worst pattern of work is probably 1 week of nights because the circadian cycle is disrupted and quality-sleep deficiency accumulates by the end of the week. As one gets older, it takes longer to recover from periods of sleep deprivation, a fact that justifies that more senior surgeons should take less on-call or night float work.

MISCELLANEOUS DESCRIPTIVE TRAITS

There are several validated descriptive traits essential to teamwork and communication. These are listed in **Table 4**, and are believed to be essential characteristics of surgical trainees.[23,24] These later become incorporated into the assessment tools for nontechnical skills.

Table 4
Essential validated nontechnical skill descriptors for surgical trainees

Skills	Median Weighting (Scale 1–5, 5 Highest)
Seeks advice when beyond limits of confidence	4
Can be trusted to carry out instruction	4
Able to communicate clearly with other staff members	3
Accepts feedback on own performance	3
Can keep on time	3
Understands other staff members' point of view	3
Delegates to others when appropriate	3
Aware of the role of other specialties	3
Able to offer constructive criticism to others	3
Reviews diagnosis and management regularly	3
Adapts quickly if problems arise	3
Knows when not to intervene	3
Decides quickly in an emergency	3
Can improvise when necessary	3
Can cope with unreasonable colleagues	2

From Paisley AM, Baldwin PJ, Paterson-Brown S. Feasibility, reliability and validity of a new assessment form for use with basic surgical trainees. Am J Surg 2001;182:29; with permission.

COGNITIVE SKILLS
Situation Awareness

Situation awareness can be defined as developing and maintaining a dynamic awareness of the situation in the OR, based on assembling data from the environment (patient, team, time, displays, equipment), understanding what they mean, and thinking ahead about what may happen next.[13] Without good situational awareness, all the other nontechnical skills struggle to succeed. There are 3 progressive levels of awareness: gathering information (level 1); interpreting the information, with experience clearly playing an important role (level 2); and projecting/anticipating future situations based on this information (level 3).[25] Ideal and adverse situations at each level are depicted in **Table 5**.

Obviously the situation can change, and adaptability is paramount during the operation. Surgeons who have good situational awareness have the ability to step back and reassess the conditions, interpret nonverbal clues in the room, and reconsider the operative strategy.

Decision Making/Anticipating Problems

This skill is defined as determining a particular course of action. Although decision making is required at many points in a patient's care (eg, whether to operate or not, how much to do, when to intervene), perhaps the one most difficult to assess is intraoperative decision making. Several models of decision making have been proposed. The first is the analytical model; this is the classic approach whereby by several options are considered but the optimal course of action is selected. The surgeon weighs the pros and cons of the different approaches and a final decision is made, often effortlessly, based on experience and situation. For example, if a nodule in a wedge resection comes back from pathology as positive for cancer, how much, if any, more lung tissue needs to be resected. Other factors come into play such as age, lung function, pathology, and location. It is estimated that surgeons use the analytical approach in 50% of cases.[26]

The next most common model is the rule-based decision, "if X then Y." This decision making process is much easier, because it is based on protocols, guidelines, or an anecdotal rule learned during training. For example, if a mediastinal lymph node comes back from pathology as metastatic disease, one would not proceed further with the lung resection.

Expert surgeons often use a recognition-primed decision style. These decisions are usually made during high stress or time pressure. They usually use the first workable decision to a problem based

Table 5
Examples of ideal and adverse behaviors for situational awareness

Element	Ideal Behavior	Adverse Behavior
Level 1: gathering information	Performs preoperative checklists All relevant imaging/tests reviewed Reviews operative plan with team Monitors ongoing blood loss Asks team for update	Arrives to OR late Asks for results at last minute Does not consider opinions or concerns of staff Fails to communicate with anesthesia team Asks staff to read notes during operation because not read preoperatively Fails to review information collected by team
Level 2: understanding information	Changes surgical plan as patient's condition changes Acts according to gathered information Reflects and discusses role of each team member Communicates priorities and plan with team	Overlooks/ignores important results Asks questions that reflect lack of understanding Misses clear issues on imaging or tests Ignores important results
Level 3: projecting and anticipating future situations	Has a contingency plan by asking for equipment potentially needed Keeps all team members informed about procedure (bleeding, when closing) Verbalizes what may be needed later in operation Cites pertinent literature on the clinical event	Overconfident maneuvers with total disregard what may go wrong Does not discuss potential problems with team Does not tell anesthesia about sudden blood loss Waits for a predicted problem to arise before responding

Adapted from Yule S, Paterson-Brown S. Surgeons' nontechnical skills. Surg Clin N Am. 2012;92(1):41; with permission.

on experience rather than work through the analytical model, because working memory space is diminished during times of stress. When trainees encounter this same situation, they have neither experience nor adequate working memory space because of the stress and complexity of the situation. For example, if the pulmonary artery branch is injured during a VATS (video-assisted thoracoscopic surgery) lobectomy, depending on the situation, would conversion to thoracotomy be prudent rather than continuing with a VATS approach.

Finally, the last method is creative decision making. This is usually the "last resort," when all other options are not possible, or have been tried and found to be inadequate. These innovative or creative decisions may work but often result in failure.

NONCOGNITIVE TRAITS
Emotional Intelligence

Some people are uncommonly good at reading body language, and are able to judge at a glance what someone is thinking and respond accordingly.

They can calm a coworker who is angry or reassure a friend who is anxious. Why are certain people so good at this? The answer may lie in one's emotional intelligence (EI). The concept of EI was introduced by Salovey and Mayer in 1990; they described it as a "type of social intelligence that captures an individual's ability to perceive, process, and regulate one's own emotions and the emotions of others".[27] It is used to influence those feelings to advantage. Individuals with higher EI are believed to perceive, process, and regulate emotions more effectively, which can lead to enhanced well-being and less emotional disturbance.

EI combines 4 different elements.[28,29] The first is self-awareness, or the ability to understand one's own feelings and behaviors. The second is self-management; about staying in situations in which one has to behave correctly. The third is social awareness; how to read the emotions and body language of others. The fourth element is relationship management; the ability to build stronger relationships with those important in one's life. Each element has corresponding traits outlined in **Table 6**. For example, if a resident gets upset

Table 6
The 4 elements of emotional intelligence and corresponding traits

Self-Awareness	Self-Management	Social Awareness	Social Skill
• Emotional self-awareness: the ability to read and understand your emotions as well as recognize their impact on work performance, relationships, and the like • Accurate self-assessment: a realistic evaluation of your strengths and limitations • Self confidence: a strong and positive sense of self-worth	• Self-control: the ability to keep disruptive emotions and impulses under control • Trustworthiness: a consistent display of honesty and integrity • Conscientiousness: the ability to manage yourself and your responsibilities • Adaptability: skill at adjusting to changing situations and overcoming obstacles • Achievement orientation: the drive to meet an internal standard of excellence • Initiative: a readiness to seize opportunities	• Empathy: skill at sensing other people's emotions, understanding their perspective, and taking an active interest in their concerns • Organizational awareness: the ability to read the currents of organizational life, build decision networks, and navigate politics • Service orientation: the ability to recognize and meet customers' needs	• Visionary leadership: the ability to take charge and inspire with a compelling vision • Influence: the ability to wield a range of persuasive tactics • Developing others: the propensity to bolster the abilities of others through feedback and guidance • Communication: skill at listening and at sending clear, convincing, and well-tuned messages • Change catalyst: proficiency in initiating new ideas and leading people in a new direction • Conflict management: the ability to deescalate disagreements and orchestrate resolutions • Building bonds: proficiency at cultivating and maintaining a web of relationships • Teamwork and collaboration: competence at promoting cooperation and building teams

From Goleman D. Leadership that gets results. Harv Bus Rev. 2000;(March-April):78-90; with permission.

when he or she is criticized, EI will help in knowing how to give feedback to which the resident will be able to respond more effectively.

Much has been written and proven about EI in the business world. EI research in the medical field is evolving and concentrated mainly in the surgical specialties. These studies on surgical residents do show that EI is a strong predictor of resident well-being and job satisfaction.[28,30] EI traits seem to be tied to leadership skills, highly valued in the surgical team-centric concept, and may be more of a useful parameter to select students, residents, and faculty in the future.[31]

Grit and Resiliency

Other noncognitive traits not associated with intellect that are difficult to quantitate relate to those skills associated with attitude, motivation, and temperament. Grit and resiliency are terms used to describe the ability to persevere through hardships to meet certain goals. Both topics have emerged in recent years as popular themes in business and are now a focus of research in medicine. Grit seems to be important for academic and professional success independent of IQ,[32] whereas resilience has been shown to be a predictor of well-being.[33] These terms are now used in academic settings, particularly with the long periods of postgraduate medical education and residency training, where there may be perceived ability (or lack thereof) to handle difficult situations and disappointments, and linked to overall life satisfaction.[34]

Grit and resiliency are often used interchangeably and related in some fashion. However, they are 2 completely different concepts. Grit is defined as having a passion and perseverance for long-term goals, and, despite episodes of adversity and setbacks, a sustained commitment carries one through to completing these endeavors.[32] Studies measuring grit in surgical training have yielded some conflicting evidence. As with other professions, grit is predictive of psychologic health[35] and may or may not lead to emotional exhaustion.[36] It remains a positive predictor of general psychologic well-being, negative for depression, with no difference between genders; those with more grit are at a lower risk for the thought of attrition from a surgical residency program,[36] which tended toward statistical significance ($P = .08$). This did not translate in true attrition, which is not an unexpected observation.

The context of resiliency can vary depending on the specific situation. Generally, it is the ability to maintain or regain mental health after experiencing adversity, with the capacity to "bounce back" after stressful or negative emotional experiences.[37] In essence, one must move on and not dwell on the past, using healthy mental strategies to handle stress and anxiety. Thus, resiliency is an integral feature of grit.

Resilience has also been broken down into 3 key concepts: a trait, a process, or an outcome.[38,39] As a trait, it is an individual characteristic with the ability to cope with stress; as a process, it is how individuals thrive in the face of adversity, recognizing that this is a dynamic process with interacting protective and risk factors; and finally as an outcome, the ability or stability for quick recovery or growth under adverse conditions. Irrespective of the perception, resiliency requires both internal factors of self-efficacy, self-control, and emotional stability and external supportive elements of personal relationships and family cohesion.[40]

There is a growing interest in research on grit and resiliency in surgical training, with data showing that both are related to predicting academic, career, and life success.[41,42] Educators and training program directors continue to evaluate what characteristics can predict success. Grit and resiliency may overlap with other noncognitive traits essential to overcome everyday obstacles and pressure; which one is most important will be difficult at best to answer, but irrespective of the element, they all will help to promote well-being and career success in and out of the OR.[36,43]

Implicit Bias

In 1990, the sentinel article by Schulman and colleagues[44] put the issue of unconscious or implicit bias at the forefront of American medicine. They concluded that the management of chest pain and need for cardiac catherization was highly influenced by gender and race. Clinical decision making relies on "physician assessment of both tangible and intangible patient characteristics, it is consequently the stage in the referral process at which race-based perceptions and biases about a patient are most likely to enter."[45]

The concept of implicit (also termed unconscious) bias rests on the belief that people act on the basis of internalized schemas of which they are unaware and thus can, and often do, engage in discriminatory behaviors without conscious intent.[46] Surgical and clinical decisions are subject to implicit stereotypes and bias. These are often in the areas of gender, race, and ethnicity. Although less studied, stereotypical views on patients' personal characteristics, such as reliability, honesty, education level, and income, may also bias medical decisions.[47]

The Association of Women Surgeons recently recommended concrete steps that can be implemented at the departmental, institutional, or national level to continue education on reducing implicit bias.[48] Irrespective of the approach to reduce implicit bias, there remains a need from one's time in medical school throughout a surgical career to encourage empathy and understanding of patients' sociocultural context to promote just and compassionate care, irrespective of race, ethnicity, gender, or other personal characteristics.

TOOLS FOR ASSESSMENT

The ACGME core competencies were developed to address primarily technical skills in the OR and communication/interpersonal skills outside the OR. To address this assessment gap, several validated tools have been developed to evaluate those intraoperative nontechnical skills of surgeons and surgical teams. These rating systems, skills assessed, and applicability are summarized in **Table 7** adapted from Sevdalis and colleagues.[49]

In addition, there has recently been a development that attempts to use cognitive assessment specifically within robotic surgery.[55] Finally, self-assessment, although informal, is the most commonly used method of evaluation and, irrespective of taxonomy, allows for self-reflection

Table 7
Assessment tools for nontechnical skills

Rating Tool	Skills Assessed	Clinical Application
Nontechnical Skills for Surgeons (NOTSS)[50]	Nontechnical skills Communication/teamwork Leadership Situation awareness Decision making	Applicable to surgical personnel only Designed for use by senior surgeons 2-day training for novice users
Nontechnical Skills, Revised (NOTECHS)[51]	Nontechnical skills Communication/interaction Situation awareness Cooperation/team skills Leadership/managerial skills Decision making	Surgical, anesthesia, and nursing personnel in the OR Can be used by both clinical and nonclinical assessors Captures performance in routine and crisis situations
Observational Teamwork Assessment for Surgery (OTAS)[52]	Clinical OR team performance Communication Cooperation/back up Coordination Leadership Team monitoring/situation awareness	Surgical, anesthesia, and nursing personnel in the OR Can be used by both clinical and nonclinical assessors Programs for novice users available
Ottawa Crisis Resource Management Global Rating Scale (Ottawa GRS)[53]	Nontechnical skills and global performance Problem solving Situational awareness Leadership Resource utilization Communication	Broadly applicable to health care teams in the acute setting Aimed at simulation-based training modules on participants' relevant skills
Oxford Nontechnical Skills (Oxford NOTECHS)[54]	Nontechnical skills Communication/interaction Situation awareness Cooperation/team skills Leadership/managerial skills Decision making	Applicable to surgical, anesthesia, and nursing personnel Can be used by both clinical and nonclinical assessors Captures performance in routine and crisis situations

Adapted from Sevdalis N, Hull L, Birnbach DJ. Improving patient safety in the operating theatre and perioperative care: obstacles, interventions, and priorities for accelerating progress. Br J Anaesth. 2012;109(S1):i9-11; with permission.

for each category and element through self-improvement.

SUMMARY

Surgery is a complex and high-risk activity. For more than a century, training from novice to expert has focused on technical skills. Nontechnical skills matter at critical stages of surgical care and should continue to be integrated into the technical curricula of residency training programs and new technology. These "alternative" skill sets are not universally trained, practiced, or assessed, but many validated tools now exist for team-based and self-assessment. Whether these qualities are achieved through "nature or nurture," acclimation to these topics is given at several levels through departments, institutions, or specialty societies. A partial table of "alternative curriculum" self-help books is presented in **Box 1**. Although many

---

Box 1
The "alternative surgical curriculum" suggested reading book list: the psychology of surgical training

Motivation/Grit/Resiliency

Daniel Pink (2009): *Drive: The Surprising Truth About What Motivates Us*

Angela Duckworth (2018): *"Grit" The Power of Passion and Perseverance*

Decision Making

Malcolm Gladwell (2005): *Blink: The Power of Thinking Without Thinking*

Zachary Shore (2008): *Blunder: Why Smart People Make Dumb Decisions*

Leadership

Jim Collins (2001): *Good to Great*

Seth Godin (2008) *Tribes*

Performance Under Stress

Paul Sullivan (2010): *Clutch*

Decision Making

Gary Klein (1999): *Sources of Power: How People Make Decisions*

Teamwork

Patrick Lencioni (2010): *The Five Dysfunctions of a Team*

Patrick Lencioni (2016): *The Ideal Team Player: How to Recognize and Cultivate the Three Essential Virtues*

Don Yaeger (2016): *Great Teams: 16 Things High Performing Organizations Do Differently*

Emotional Intelligence

Goldman D (1995). *Emotional Intelligence: Why It Matters More Than IQ*

Goldman D (2015): *HBR's 10 Must Reads on Emotional Intelligence*

Travis Bradberry and Jean Greaves (2009): *Emotional Intelligence 2.0*

Daniel Goldman, Richard Boyatzis, and Annie McKee (2013): *Primal Leadership: Unleashing the Power of Emotional Intelligence*

Implicit Bias

Mahzarin Banaji and Anthony Greenwald (2013): *Blindspot: Hidden Biases of Good People*

of these traits tie into leadership and competency in the OR, ultimately they can affect one's personal life and well-being, and thus should be a primary focus at a time when resiliency in surgery is challenged.

REFERENCES

1. Helmreich RL, Schaefer HG. Team performance in the operating room. In: Bogner M, editor. Human error in medicine. Hillsdale (NJ): Lawrence Erlbaum Associates; 1994. p. 225–53.
2. Rogers SO Jr, Gawande AA, Kwaan M, et al. Analysis of surgical errors in closed malpractice claims at 4 liability insurers. Surgery 2006;140(1):25–33.
3. British Medical Association, National Patient Safety Agency, NHS Modernisation Agency. Safe handover: safe patients, Guid Clin Handover Clin Manag. 2005. Available at: http://www.saferhealthcare.org.uk/IHI/Products/Publications/.
4. Institute of Medicine. Crossing the quality chasm: a new health system for the 21st century. Available at: http://www.iom.edu/Reports/2001/Crossing-the-Quality-Chasm-A-New-Health-System-for-the-21st-Century.Aspx. Accessed March 27, 2019.
5. Roughton V, Severs M. The junior doctor handover: current practices and future expectations. J R Coll Physicians Lond 1996;30:213–4.
6. Todkode M, O'Riordan B, Bartholmes L. That's all I got handed over: missed opportunities and opportunity for near misses in Wales. BMJ 2006;332:610.
7. Todkode M, O'Riordan B, Bartholmes L. Near-misses and missed opportunities: poor patient handover in general surgery. Ann R Coll Surg Engl 2008;90:96–8.
8. Nagpal K, Abboudi M, Manchanda C, et al. Improving postoperative handover: a prospective observational study. Am J Surg 2013;206(4): 494–501.
9. Carthey J, de Leval MR, Reason JT. Understanding excellence in complex, dynamic medical domains. In: Proceedings of the International Ergonomics Association and Human Factors Society triennial conference. Santa Monica (CA): The Human Factors and Ergonomic Society Press; 2000. p. 136–9.
10. Maykel JA. Leadership in surgery. Clin Colon Rectal Surg 2013;26(4):254–8.
11. Chen XP, Williams RG, Sanfey HA, et al. A taxonomy of surgeons' guiding behaviors in the operating room. Am J Surg 2015;209(1):15–20.
12. Stone JL, Aveling E-L, Frean M, et al. Effective leadership of surgical teams: a mixed methods study of surgeon behaviors and functions. Ann Thorac Surg 2017;104(2):530–7.
13. Yule S, Paterson-Brown S. Surgeons' non-technical skills. Surg Clin North Am 2012;92:37–50.
14. Wray RC. The dream fades. Plast Reconstr Surg 1983;71(1):107–8.
15. Balch CM, Shanafelt T. Combating stress and burnout in surgical practice: a review. Thorac Surg Clin 2011;21(3):417–30.
16. Arora S, Sevdalis N, Nestel D, et al. The impact of stress on surgical performance: a systematic review of the literature. Surgery 2010;147:318–30.
17. Shanafelt TD, Balch CM, Bechamps GJ, et al. Burnout and career satisfaction among American surgeons. Ann Surg 2009;250(3):463–71.
18. Squiers JJ, Lobdell KW, Fann JI, et al. Physician burnout: are we treating the symptoms instead of the disease? Ann Thorac Surg 2017;104(4):1117–22.
19. Block L, Habicht R, Wu AW, et al. In the wake of the 2003 and 2011 duty hours regulations, how do internal medicine interns spend their time? J Gen Intern Med 2013;28:1042–7.
20. Chung RS, Ahmed N. How surgical residents spend their training time: the effect of a goal-oriented work style on efficiency and work satisfaction. Arch Surg 2007;142:249–52.
21. Woolhandler W, Himmelstein DU. Administrative work consumes one-sixth of U.S. physicians' working hours and lowers their career satisfaction. Int J Health Serv 2014;44:635–42.

22. Lockley SW, Cronin JW, Evans EE, et al. Harvard work hours, health and safety effect of reducing interns' weekly work hours on sleep and attentional failures. N Engl J Med 2004;351(18):1829–37.

23. Baldwin PJ, Paisley AM, Paterson-Brown S. Consultant surgeons' opinions of the skills required of basic surgical trainees. Br J Surg 1999;86:1078–82.

24. Paisley AM, Baldwin PJ, Paterson-Brown S. Feasibility, reliability and validity of a new assessment form for use with basic surgical trainees. Am J Surg 2001;182:24–9.

25. Endsley M, Garland D. Situation awareness. Analysis and measurement. Mahwah (NJ): Lawrence Erlbaum Associates; 2000.

26. Pauley K, Flin R, Yule S, et al. Surgeons' intraoperative decision making and risk management. Am J Surg 2011;202(4):375–81.

27. Salovey P, Mayer JD. Emotional intelligence. Imagin Cogn Pers 1990;9:185 211.

28. Goleman D. Leadership that gets results. Harvard Business Review 2000;78 90.

29. Lin DT, Liebert CA, Tran J, et al. Emotional intelligence as a predictor of resident well-being. J Am Coll Surg 2016;223(2):352–8.

30. Hollis RH, Theiss LM, Gullick AA, et al. Emotional intelligence in surgery is associated with resident job satisfaction. J Surg Res 2017;209:178–83.

31. Erdman MK, Bonaroti A, Provenzano G, et al. Street smarts and a scalpel: emotional intelligence in surgical education. J Surg Educ 2017;74(2):277–85.

32. Duckworth AL, Peterson C, Matthews MD, et al. Grit: perseverance and passion for long-term goals. J Pers Soc Psychol 2007;92(6):1087–101.

33. Epstein RM, Krasner MS. Physician resilience: what it means, why it matters, and how to promote it. Acad Med 2013;88(3):301–3.

34. Clark KN, Malecki CK. Academic Grit Scale: psychometric properties and associations with achievement and life satisfaction. J Sch Psychol 2019;72: 49–66.

35. Salles A, Cohen GL, Mueller CM. The relationship between grit and resident well-being. Am J Surg 2014;207(2):251–4.

36. Salles A, Lin D, Liebert C, et al. Grit as a predictor of risk of attrition in surgical residency. Am J Surg 2017;213(2):288–91.

37. Tugade MM, Fredrickson BL. Resilient individuals use positive emotions to bounce back from negative emotional experiences. J Pers Soc Psychol 2004; 86(2):320–33.

38. Fletcher D, Sarkar M. Psychological resilience: a review and critique of definitions, concepts, and theory. Eur Psychol 2013;18:12.

39. Ng R, Chahine S, Lanting S, et al. Unpacking the literature on stress and resiliency: a narrative review focused on learners in the operating room. J Surg Educ 2019;76(2):343–53.

40. Windle G. What is resilience? A review and concept analysis. Rev Clin Gerontol 2011;21:152–69.

41. Howe A, Smajdor A, Stöckl A. Towards an understanding of resilience and its relevance to medical training. Med Educ 2012;46(4):349–56.

42. Hammond DA. Grit: an important characteristic in learners. Curr Pharm Teach Learn 2016;9(1):1–3.

43. Burkhart RA, Tholey RM, Guinto D, et al. Grit: a marker of residents at risk for attrition? Surgery 2014;155(6):1014–22.

44. Schulman KA, Berlin JA, Harless W, et al. The effect of race and sex on physicians' recommendations for cardiac catheterization. N Engl J Med 1999;340(8): 618–26.

45. Einbinder LC, Schulman KA. The effect of race on the referral process for invasive cardiac procedures. Med Care Res Rev 2000;57(Suppl 1):162–80.

46. Pritlove C, Juando-Prats C, Ala-leppilampi K, et al. The good, the bad and the ugly about implicit bias. Lancet 2019;393:502–4.

47. Santry HP, Wren SM. The role of unconscious bias in surgical safety and outcomes. Surg Clin North Am 2012;92(1):137–51.

48. DiBrito SR, Lopez CM, Jones C, et al. Reducing implicit bias: association of women surgeons #HeforShe task force best practice recommendations. J Am Coll Surg 2019;228(3):303–9.

49. Sevdalis N, Hull L, Birnbach DJ. Improving patient safety in the operating theatre and perioperative care: obstacles, interventions, and priorities for accelerating progress. Br J Anaesth 2012;109: i3 16.

50. Steinemann S, Berg B, DiTullio A, et al. Assessing teamwork in the trauma bay: introduction of a modified "NOTECHS " scale for trauma. Am J Surg 2012; 203:69–75.

51. Sevdalis N, Davis RE, Koutantji M, et al. Reliability of a revised NOTECHS scale for use in surgical teams. Am J Surg 2008;196:184–90.

52. Hull L, Arora S, Kassab E, et al. Observational teamwork assessment for surgery (OTAS): content validation and tool refinement. J Am Coll Surg 2011; 212:234–43.

53. Kim J, Neilipovitz D, Cardinal P, et al. A pilot study using high-fidelity simulation to formally evaluate performance in the resuscitation of critically ill patients: the University of Ottawa Critical Care Medicine, High-Fidelity Simulation, and Crisis Resource Management I Study. Crit Care Med 2006;34: 2167–74.

54. Mishra A, Catchpole K, McCulloch P. The Oxford NOTECHS System: reliability and validity of a tool for measuring teamwork behaviour in the operating theatre. Qual Saf Health Care 2009;18:104–8.

55. Guru KA, Esfahani ET, Raza SJ, et al. Cognitive skills assessment during robot-assisted surgery: separating wheat from chaff. BJU Int 2014;115:166–74.

Deliberate Practice and the Emerging Roles of Simulation in Thoracic Surgery

Phillip G. Rowse, MD*, Joseph A. Dearani, MD

KEYWORDS

- Deliberate practice • Simulation • Cardiac surgery • Thoracic surgery

KEY POINTS

- Deliberate practice and surgical simulation foster self-regulated learning behaviors.
- Surgical skill acquisition through simulation in cardiothoracic surgery is transferrable.
- Faculty supervision and feedback remain critical elements in deliberate practice.

INTRODUCTION

Excellence in cardiothoracic surgery is anything but mundane. Or is it? In the early 1980s, Chambliss[1] described the mundanity of excellence as, "consistent superiority of performance." He came to this discovery by stratifying the training habits of competitive swimmers wherein he observed superlative performance by world-class Olympic swimmers to be a confluence of dozens of small learned skills carefully drilled into habit by attentive focus and perfect practice. Similarly, excellence in cardiothoracic surgery requires assimilation and mastery of hundreds of fundamental technical skills that when independently examined may elementally appear mundane, yet when integrated and choreographed within an operation reflect the product of an elite surgeon.

Simulation in cardiothoracic surgery has come into spotlight as surgical educators have used this platform like the "Olympic training pool" wherein perfect practice and repetition in a safe and structured environment can be drilled into habit with constructive feedback. Ericsson[2,3] defines this method of training as deliberate practice (DP), which actually has 4 core components: it identifies a specific goal(s) for performance improvement, requires intense focus, provides immediate feedback by an expert, and is designed to stretch an individual's capacity to function with increasing task complexity. This review provides a focused synthesis of evidence regarding simulation-based training and DP as a whole and within the specialty of cardiothoracic surgery.

THE CHALLENGE

Apprenticeship teaching in the operating room is currently the most common and widely practiced method for surgical instruction. It is also, perhaps, most variable in terms of experience gained as a result of varied levels of staff commitment to education. When I was in training, this letter by Dearani[4] candidly articulated the expectations he had for all residents when starting on service with him. The usefulness of this "letter" proved face-value dividends in terms of amplifying our experiences as we internalized the objectives and put them to the test. Setting and reviewing service guidelines that encompass preoperative, day of surgery, postoperative care, and general pearls of success is but a simple way surgical staff can instill trust and confidence in young trainees and elevate them to a higher level of functioning. In short, it is a straightforward way to mentor the apprentice.

Disclosure Statement: The authors have nothing to disclose.
Department of Cardiovascular Surgery, Mayo Clinic, 200 First Street Southwest, Rochester, MN 55905, USA
* Corresponding author.
E-mail address: Rowse.Phillip@mayo.edu

Thorac Surg Clin 29 (2019) 303–309
https://doi.org/10.1016/j.thorsurg.2019.03.007
1547-4127/19/© 2019 Elsevier Inc. All rights reserved.

Surgical instruction in the operating room may not be the most valuable place to initially learn fundamental technical skills in cardiothoracic surgery as there is often a low tolerance for learning inefficiency, it complies poorly with the core principles of DP, is time sensitive, and does not adequately ensure exposure to all intraoperative complications, including crisis management. In addition, staff surgeons are under enormous pressure for individual perfection in light of patient safety concerns, quality metrics, public reporting, and hospital transparencies, not to mention the surplus of higher risk surgical patients being referred for more complex procedures.[5–7] Furthermore, a recent study of cardiothoracic residents by Stephens and colleagues[8] identified "public scrutiny" of surgical outcomes as a leading issue perceived by residents that adversely affects the quality of training. Indeed, the former "see one, do one, teach one," training model is now obsolete.

On the other hand, cardiothoracic surgical residents and fellows are challenged with the need to acquire safe and proficient fundamental technical skills as well as the necessary cognitive growth and refinement in clinical judgment needed to market themselves as capable surgeons. This maturation process, leading to board eligibility by the American Board of Thoracic Surgery (ABTS), is expected to be accomplished over a traditional ("5 + 2" or "5 + 3"), joint ("4 + 3"), or integrated (I-6) program amid an overall national reduction in resident cardiothoracic operative volume following the inception of the 80-hour work week in 2003.[9–11] In addition, a trend of increased failure on the ABTS board examination may yet be another unintended consequence of duty hour restrictions.[12]

A NATIONAL EFFORT IN CARDIOTHORACIC SIMULATION

The role of simulation-based training and purposeful DP as a supplement to apprenticeship teaching is gaining favor in all disciplines of surgery, including cardiothoracic education. Under the auspices of the Thoracic Surgery Directors Association (TSDA), a national effort to provide annual structured simulation training in cardiothoracic surgery was established in 2008. This 3-day simulation curriculum, termed "boot camp," was designed for all incoming first-year traditional and fourth-year integrated cardiothoracic surgical residents in the United States. Junior-level trainees were likely selected for this workshop, as simulation studies indicate a more profound benefit of surgical simulation among more junior-

level trainees.[13,14] In accordance with the core components of DP, the TSDA-driven boot camp established goals for resident performance improvement in 5 areas of cardiothoracic surgery: cardiopulmonary bypass and cannulation, coronary anastomosis, bronchoscopy/mediastinoscopy, anatomic pulmonary resection, and aortic valve replacement. Didactic sessions are led by expert faculty surgeons followed by hands-on high-fidelity simulator and wet laboratory training, which provide an intense focus-driven learning opportunity designed to stretch residents to learn and perform outside their current level of comfort and ability. Each participant is evaluated and given immediate feedback during the simulation sessions. This national scale effort has become a critical element of simulation-based learning for more than a third of incoming cardiothoracic surgical trainees for the past 10 years. All participants have highly rated the overall learning experience and the volume of simulation literature produced from this academic work lends further credence to a modular approach to technical skill acquisition.[15–17] Boot camp attendees also have been found to be 2 times more likely to pass their ABTS board examination than those who did not attend.[18] Furthermore, although the primary objective of boot camp is the advancement of fundamental knowledge and skill through simulation for residents, Fann and colleagues[19] pointed out that it has also benefited academic surgeons at the faculty level in 2 concrete ways: (1) it has helped broaden acceptance of simulation training and (2) it has refined surgical teaching through creation of an educator course that has helped nearly 100 faculty members to date improve teaching behaviors and skills that may further enhance learning outcomes for cardiothoracic trainees.

The TSDA acknowledges that boot camp is not the "silver bullet" of cardiothoracic surgical simulation education. In fact, one of the main perceived pitfalls of boot camp is the concern of whether or not the knowledge and skills inculcated by a single "massed practice" session without longitudinal follow-up are actually translatable to clinical practice. In other words, do simulation-acquired surgical skills transfer to the operating room? The answer is, "YES!" Several randomized studies performed in the days of simulation infancy within the specialty of surgery have demonstrated a direct association between simulation training in the laboratory setting and improved performance in the operating room along with a decrease in operative time and intraoperative error.[20–23] More recently, a review of 27 randomized comparative studies have corroborated the finding that surgical simulation participants who reached procedural proficiency on a simulator perform better in the clinical environment than their non–simulation-trained counterparts.[24] Nonetheless, the direct correlation of such improvements in intraoperative errors, operative time, or performance in terms of clinical relevancy to the patient (ie, complications or length of stay) has not been clearly established. Or has it? Simulation-based training in colonoscopy has documented improvement in patient comfort during the procedure[25]; a reduction in mortality has been documented after implementation of simulation-based cardiopulmonary resuscitation curricula in the intensive care unit[26]; and a reduction in central venous catheter–related complications has been observed with adoption and widespread implementation of simulation training.[27] Furthermore, a randomized study by Zendejas and colleagues[28] objectively revealed a direct patient benefit with reduced intraoperative complications and earlier hospital dismissal following participation in a simulated inguinal herniorrhaphy curriculum. A common denominator identified in many of these clinical relevancy simulation studies is the model of DP with continued effort until a predefined level of performance associated with "mastery" was achieved. Who then are the direct beneficiaries of simulation? Our patients and our trainees!

SIMULATION-BASED TRAINING AND DELIBERATE PRACTICE

To become an expert performer in any given area (ie, music, sports, entertainment, medicine) it is necessary to first identify reproducibly superior performance in the real world and then capture and reproduce that performance ideally with standardized tasks that can be studied and practiced in a laboratory-type setting. When this type of repetitive training is supervised and guided by an expert teacher, it is called DP, a concept first introduced in 1993 by Ericsson and colleagues.[2] As mentioned previously, DP must contain specific practice activities or training tasks that align with desired training goals set and monitored by the student and expert teacher. The student must practice with full concentration and receive immediate feedback with gradual improvement in structure and complexity of practice.

The literature supporting this method of simulation training including the value of independent practice in cardiothoracic surgery is mounting. Fann and colleagues[29] studied the outcomes of simulated coronary anastomosis by cardiothoracic residents on a beating heart following instruction and low-fidelity task trainer practice at home. They discovered a 15% to 20% reduction

in task completion time on a beating heart model with improvement in performance ratings following independent home practice. Unfortunately, not all residents improved, which identifies 2 important limitations in surgical simulation and DP: (1) a "ceiling effect" with regard to simulator usefulness, and (2) a "plateau effect" with regard to surgical trainee performance improvement.

A recent meta-analysis of 17 simulation-based bronchoscopic training studies using the fundamentals of DP found bronchoscopic simulation effective and transferable to patient care in the areas of bronchoscopic inspection, foreign-body removal, endobronchial ultrasound, trans-bronchial needle aspiration, and rigid bronchoscopy.[30] In the meta-analysis, performance assessments and feedback were found to be most constructive and useful to the trainee if a validated assessment tool (ie, objective structured assessment of technical skills) was used.[31] Furthermore, longer structured training was found to be more valuable than self-practice in this particular study. No clear advantage in the type of bronchoscopic training instrument was found, although a trend favored animal models and low-cost, low-fidelity mannequins over virtual reality simulators. Although simulation-based training was found to be clearly effective, the optimal design of such instruction to guide expert bronchoscopic teachers regarding number and sequence of training tasks was lacking.

Helder and colleagues[32] showed the value of using a Web-based instructional video on aortic anastomosis to support DP at home with a low-cost, low-fidelity task simulator. In that study, medical students were shown to have the greatest benefit from using an online video curriculum in conjunction with the accompanying "take home" simulator when compared with surgical and cardiothoracic residents on a high-fidelity porcine posttest assessment. This finding raises an interesting question regarding appropriate timing for simulating fundamental skills in cardiothoracic surgery. Should we begin training young medical students long before formal matriculation into cardiothoracic residency? Additionally, some evidence suggests that early surgical exposure may influence medical students' choice of careers.[33] In addition, an Internet-based, audiovisual (AV) skills curriculum is a stirring idea that may be a useful vehicle to disseminate extraordinary surgeon-educator knowledge and skill around the globe with limitless reaching potential with relatively little upfront effort by the expert surgeon (ie, create an educational "how-to" video). A recent innovative study of 20 surgical procedures disseminated via an online AV simulation curriculum (accompanied with low-cost low-fidelity simulators) was found to support individualized DP and was readily received by millennial learners.[34]

As technical complexity of cardiothoracic surgical procedures increases, DP and simulation will become more important for trainees. Surgical management of congenital heart diseases and performance of minimally invasive esophagectomy are 2 examples of technically demanding fields with steep learning curves that impose considerable learning challenges on trainees and surgeon mentors. Mavroudis and colleagues[35] recently explored the feasibility of simulating a variety of index congenital heart operations using high-fidelity simulation (ie, a neonatal porcine model). In this study, the principles of DP were used with focused effort in practicing and performing the following procedures: Norwood procedure, arterial switch, ventricular septal defect and atrial septal defect closure, Ross procedure, systemic pulmonary artery shunt procedures, tricuspid repair, transmediastinal coarctectomy with extended end-to-end anastomosis, right ventricle to pulmonary artery conduit, and Tetralogy of Fallot repair. Fabian and colleagues[36] likewise used a high-fidelity porcine model (ex vivo) combined with a thoracoscopic task trainer to help general thoracic surgical residents learn and deliberately practice intrathoracic anastomoses, thereby simulating a critical step in minimally invasive Ivor Lewis esophagectomy.

Both of these studies demonstrated the feasibility of simulating and mentoring trainee performance of technically demanding operations in a high-fidelity simulated learning environment. Consequently, trainee confidence, skill, and overall education were enhanced by making and correcting mistakes with guided mentorship in a safe and controlled simulation milieu. An obvious disadvantage of using high-fidelity porcine sim models is the considerable cost and inability to use the model continuously over time. Virtual 3D printing with hydrogel material is a potential alternative to animal models that preserves fidelity and even enables patient-specific abnormalities to be examined and practiced beforehand. This may be extraordinarily useful in the training environment, as prior difficult cases may be repeatedly used for resident education. Hermsen and colleagues[37] have successfully presented the idea of printing, planning, practicing, and performing septal myectomy for hypertrophic cardiomyopathy using the platform of 3-dimensional (3D) printing to improve surgical training of a traditionally difficult-to-teach operation.

Despite important work on model development (low-cost/low-fidelity, animal, virtual reality, and 3D) there is also needed understanding within the realm of curricular development. What kind of DP makes perfect? In other words, does it matter the ways in which the training of surgical residents is delivered (ie, how, what, when, and how often?). We have previously introduced the methodology of "massed practice," which is practice delivered in continuous blocks of time with little or no rest in-between (ie, boot camp). In contrast, "distributed practice," follows the pattern of practice interspersed with periods of rest. There is good evidence within the fields of psychology and athletics that supports distributed practice over massed practice in terms of motor skill acquisition and retention.[38–40] Recently, surgical educators have begun testing these theories to see how well they apply to surgical skill acquisition.[41–46] For example, Moulton and colleagues[47] evaluated 38 junior surgical residents in performance of microvascular anastomosis after randomly being assigned to either massed practice (1 day) or distributed (weekly) practice regimens. Performances were evaluated before, after, and 1 month after training. Although both groups showed improvement in microvascular anastomotic skill, the distributed practice group performed significantly better on retention testing and on outcome measures (ie, time, number of hand movements, checklist score, expert global ratings, and final product). Thus, despite a greater logistical challenge, focusing DP efforts with periods of rest should be the primary goal of any surgical skills curricula.

Verrier[48] reported "mindset determines how we think, grit determines if we succeed, DP should determine how we train, and coaching is essential to performance." Unfortunately, not all elite faculty surgeons are expert teachers or coaches. A recent study by Fann and colleagues[19] sought to understand how teaching behaviors in cardiothoracic surgery contribute to simulation-based learning. Teaching behaviors of faculty participating in boot camp were initially evaluated (by residents and faculty) and then reevaluated by faculty 3 months later. Overall, simulation-based training at boot camp was perceived by residents to be associated with positive teaching behaviors. Faculty ratings of themselves at boot camp revealed that they did not routinely use many of the teaching behaviors demonstrated at boot camp, indicating room for improvement in the clinical realm. At 3 months after boot camp, reassessment of faculty indicated they were implementing and improving particular teaching behaviors; however, these behaviors were still more effectively observed within the simulation environment than in the clinical setting. Hence, although trainee participation in the cardiothoracic operating room will always be metered, engagement of simulation by faculty may correlate with introspective changes in teaching.

Expert faculty members fulfill a key role in DP: they provide constructive and directive feedback to the learner. This is critically important during the early phases of task repetition and performance, as it can aid successive refinement of the task or technique being learned. Over time, however, the master teacher in any domain will help the student develop his or her own mental representations of perfect performance, such that the student can eventually take on most of the teacher's role, and eventually evaluate his or her own structured performance, provide his or her own critical feedback, and eventually design his or her own practice goals. In essence, the trainee becomes a self-regulated learner. In addition, Dearani and colleagues[49] reported mastery of DP as a key element in the acquisition of improvisational surgical skills, as preparation for improvisation infers attainment of a high level of deliberateness. With that in mind, DP can therefore improve accuracy and operative efficiency with the staff surgeon functioning as the early catalyst.

The successful cardiothoracic surgeon of tomorrow will indelibly possess the following 5 critical traits depicted in **Fig. 1**: grit, intellect, critical thinking, judgment, and technical ability.[50] Duckworth[51] defines grit as having more stamina than intensity, possessing a high degree of passion and perseverance (in spite of obstacles), and a resistance to complacency. We believe the rigorous completion of a 6-year to 8-year cardiothoracic surgical residency is correlative with becoming an early "grit" paragon, as grit is somewhat inherent among all surgeons. The written ABTS qualifying examination is structured to measure "intellect" as well as "critical-thinking" skills

(ie, is the trainee well versed in cardiothoracic diseases, including their surgical management?). Likewise, the oral ABTS certifying examination further evaluates "critical thinking" as well as "judgment" (ie, has the trainee inculcated safe surgical practices, including the careful management of unexpected or complex problems?). But what about "technical ability"? Currently there is no required formal or summative assessment of a trainee's technical skill and ability at the completion of cardiothoracic surgical training. Although this may yet be part of the ABTS certifying process in the future as recommended by some experts,[35] the astute trainee of today might presently ask, "am I doing the most I can do on my own to demonstrate my commitment to self-improvement and surgical readiness?" Using simulation as a potential examination method for ABTS board certification is a provocative and even intimidating idea; however, the value of simulation including the role of DP in skill acquisition (or surgical ability), and overall performance critique cannot be overemphasized. In a recent article by Han and Patrick,[52] the importance of independent and DP outside of the operating room was cited as a "necessary strategy" and "stand-alone ethical imperative" within our current duty-hour–restricted era of training. Furthermore, Dearani and Stulak[50] conclusively affirm the quest to improve performance is mandated on a determination to adapt, change, persist, and "practice" at *every level* during the course of a surgical career. In short, the maturation of surgical ability within our current culture must be a deliberate effort that requires both mental conditioning and resilience.

SUMMARY

Although many aspects of simulation in cardiothoracic surgery remain to be developed, DP and simulation within our specialty has been shown to improve the performer's ability to plan, assess, evaluate performance, increase technical skill, and provide safer care for patients.[2,49] In the current era of duty hour limitations and societal focus on cardiothoracic surgical outcomes, we believe an immersion in simulation with guided mentorship focused on the principles of DP will be the framework for trainees to become self-regulated learners whereby excellence eventually becomes a mundane experience.

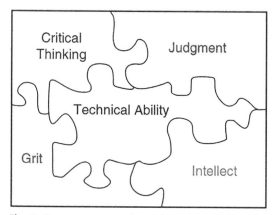

Fig. 1. Surgeon success depends on integration of 5 important variables. Technical ability is 1 element, and it can be improved with independent and DP. (*From* Dearani JA, Stulak JM. In surgical training, practice makes...almost perfect. J Thorac Cardiovasc Surg. 2018 Sep 4. In press; with permission.)

REFERENCES

1. Chambliss DF. The mundanity of excellence: an ethnographic report on stratification and Olympic swimmers. Socio Theor 1989;7(1):70–86.

2. Ericsson KA, Krampe RT, Tesch-Romer C. The role of deliberate practice in the acquisition of expert performance. Psychol Rev 1993;100:363–406.

3. Ericsson KA. Deliberate practice and the acquisition and maintenance of expert performance in medicine and related domains. Acad Med 2004;79:S70–81.

4. Dearani JA. A letter to the resident starting my service.... World J Pediatr Congenit Heart Surg 2018; 9(4):381–2.

5. Reznick RK, MacRae H. Teaching surgical skills—changes in the wind. N Engl J Med 2006;355: 2664–9.

6. Hutter MM, Kellogg KC, Ferguson CM, et al. The impact of the 80-hour resident workweek on surgical residents and attending surgeons. Ann Surg 2006; 243(6):864–71.

7. Shahian DM, Edwards FH, Jacobs JP, et al. Public reporting of cardiac surgery performance: part 1—history, rationale, consequences. Ann Thorac Surg 2011;92(3 Suppl):S2–11.

8. Stephens EH, Cornwell LD, Simpson KH, et al. Perceptions and expectations of cardiothoracic residents and attending surgeons. J Surg Res 2012; 177(2):e45–52.

9. Damadi A, Davis AT, Saxe A, et al. ACGME duty-hour restrictions decrease resident operative volume: a 5-year comparison at an ACGME-accredited university general surgery residency. J Surg Educ 2007;64(5):256–9.

10. Philbert I, Friedmann P, Williams WT. New requirements for resident duty hours. JAMA 2002;288(9):1112–4.

11. Fletcher KE, Davis SQ, Underwood W. Systematic review: effects of resident work hours on patient safety. Ann Intern Med 2004;141(11):851–7.

12. Mofatt-Bruce SD, Ross P, Williams TE Jr. American Board of Thoracic Surgery examination: fewer graduates, more failures. J Thorac Cardiovasc Surg 2014;147(5):1464–9.

13. Wenzel KR, Matsumoto ED, Hamstra SJ, et al. Teaching technical skills: training on a simple, inexpensive, and portable model. Plast Reconstr Surg 2002;109:258–64.

14. Grober ED, Hamstra SJ, Wanzel KR, et al. The educational impact of bench model fidelity on the acquisition of technical skill. Ann Surg 2004;240:374–81.

15. Macfie RC, Webel AD, Nesbitt JC, et al. Boot camp simulator training in open hilar dissection in early cardiothoracic surgical residency. Ann Thorac Surg 2014;97(1):161–6.

16. Fann JI, Calhoon JH, Carpenter AJ, et al. Simulation in coronary artery anastomosis early in cardiothoracic surgical residency training: the boot camp experience. J Thorac Cardiovasc Surg 2010; 139(5):1275–81.

17. Hicks GL Jr, Gangemi J, Angona RE, et al. Cardiopulmonary bypass simulation at the boot camp. J Thorac Cardiovasc Surg 2011;141(1):284–92.

18. Available at: https://www.tsda.org/education/boot-camp/. Accessed April 16, 2019.

19. Fann JI, Sullivan ME, Skeff KM, et al. Teaching behaviors in the cardiac surgery simulation environment. J Thorac Cardiovasc Surg 2013;145(1):45–53.

20. Van Sickle KR, Ritter EM, Baghai M, et al. Prospective, randomized, double-blind trial of curriculum-based training for intracorporeal suturing and knot tying. J Am Coll Surg 2008;207(4):560–8.

21. Larse CR, Soerensen JL, Grantcharov TP, et al. Effect of virtual reality training on laparoscopic surgery: randomized controlled trial. BMJ 2009;338: b1802.

22. Seymour NE, Gallagher AG, Roman SA, et al. Virtual reality training improves operating room performance: results of a randomized, double-blinded study. Ann Surg 2002;236(4):458–63.

23. Korndorffer JR Jr, Dunne JB, Sierra R, et al. Simulator training for laparoscopic suturing using performance goals translates to the operating room. J Am Coll Surg 2005;201(1):23–9.

24. Dawe SR, Pena GN, Windosr JA, et al. Systematic review of skills transfer after surgical simulation-based training. Br J Surg 2014;101:1063–76.

25. Sedlack RE, Kolars JC, Alexander JA. Computer simulation training enhances patient comfort during endoscopy. Clin Gastroenterol Hepatol 2004;2(4):348–52.

26. Andreatta P, Saxton E, Thompson M, et al. Simulation-based mock codes significantly correlate with improved pediatric patient cardiopulmonary arrest survival rates. Pediatr Crit Care Med 2011;12(1):33–8.

27. Barsuk JH, McGaghie WC, Cohen ER, et al. Simulation-based mastery learning reduces complications during central venous catheter insertion in a medical intensive care unit. Crit Care Med 2009;37(10): 2697–701.

28. Zendejas B, Cook DA, Bingener J, et al. Simulation-based mastery learning improves patient outcomes in laparoscopic inguinal hernia repair: a randomized controlled trial. Ann Surg 2011;254(3):502–9.

29. Fann JI, Caffarelli AD, Georgette G. Improvement in coronary anastomosis with cardiac surgery simulation. J Thorac Cardiovasc Surg 2008;136(6): 1486–91.

30. Kennedy CC, Maldonado F, Cook DA. Simulation-based bronchoscopy training: systematic review and meta-analysis. Chest 2013;144(1):183–92.

31. Martin JA, Regehr G, Reznick R, et al. Objective structured assessment of technical skill (OSATS) for surgical residents. Br J Surg 1997;84:273–8.

32. Helder MR, Rowse PG, Ruparel RK, et al. Basic cardiac surgery skills on sale for $22.50: an aortic anastomosis simulation curriculum. Ann Thorac Surg 2016;101(1):316–22.

33. Erzurum VZ, Obermeyer RJ, Fescher A, et al. What influences medical students' choice of surgical careers. Surgery 2000;128:253–6.

34. AlJamal YN, Ali SM, Ruparel RK, et al. The rationale for combining an online audiovisual curriculum with simulation to better educate general surgery trainees. Surgery 2004;156(3):723–8.

35. Mavroudis CD, Mavroudis C, Jacobs JP. Simulation and deliberate practice in a porcine model for congenital heart surgery training. Ann Thorac Surg 2018;105(2):637–43.

36. Fabian T, Glotzer OS, Bakhos CT. Construct validation: simulation of thoracoscopic intrathoracic anastomosis. JSLS 2015;19(2) [pii:e2015.00001].

37. Hermsen JL, Burke TM, Selsar SP, et al. Scan, plan, practice, perform: development and use of a patient-specific 3-dimensional printed model in adult cardiac surgery. J Thorac Cardiovasc Surg 2017;153(1):132–40.

38. Lee TD, Genovese ED. Distribution of practice in motor skill acquisition: learning and performance effects reconsidered. Res Q Exerc Sport 1988;59: 277–87.

39. Schmidt RA, Bjork RA. New conceptualization of practice: common principles in three paradigms suggest new concepts for training. Psych Sci 1992;3:207–18.

40. Donovan JJ, Radosevich DJ. A meta-analytic review of the distribution of practice effect: now you see it, now you don't. J Appl Psychol 1999;84:795–805.

41. Mackay S, Morgan P, Datta V, et al. Practice distribution in procedural skills training: a randomized controlled trial. Surg Endosc 2002;16:957–61.

42. Rogers DA, Regehr G, Howdieshell TR, et al. The impact of external feedback on computer-assisted learning for surgical technical skill training. Am J Surg 2000;179:341–3.

43. Rogers DA, Regehr G, Yeh KA, et al. Computer-assisted learning versus a lecture and feedback seminar for teaching a basic surgical technical skill. Am J Surg 1998;175:508–10.

44. Dubrowski A, Xeroulis G. Computer-based video instructions for acquisition of technical skills. J Vis Commun Med 2005;28:150–5.

45. Dubrowski A, Backstein D, Abughaduma R, et al. The influence of practice schedules in the learning of a complex bone-plating surgical task. Am J Surg 2005;190:359–63.

46. Dubrowski A, Backstein D. The contributions of kinesiology to surgical education. J Bone Joint Surg Am 2004;86:2778–81.

47. Moulton CA, Dubrowski A, MacRae H, et al. Teaching surgical skills: what kind of practice makes perfect? Ann Surg 2006;244:400–9.

48. Vorrier ED. The elite athlete, the master surgeon. J Am Coll Surg 2017;224(3):225–35.

49. Dearani JA, Gold M, Leibovich BC, et al. The role of imaging, deliberate practice, structure, and improvisation in approaching surgical perfection. J Thorac Cardiovasc Surg 2017;154(4):1329–36.

50. Dearani JA, Stulak JM. In surgical training, practice makes…almost perfect. J Thorac Cardiovasc Surg 2018. https://doi.org/10.1016/j.jtcvs.2018.08.055.

51. Duckworth A. Grit. How grity are you?. In: Grit: the power of passion and perseverance. New York: Scribner; 2016. p. 56.

52. Han JJ, Patrick WL. See one—practice—do one—practice—teach one—practice: the importance of practicing outside of the operating room in surgical training. J Thorac Cardiovasc Surg 2019;157(2): 671–7.

Teaching, Mentorship, and Coaching in Surgical Education

Jules Lin, MD*, Rishindra M. Reddy, MD

KEYWORDS

• Teaching • Surgical coaching • Mentorship

KEY POINTS

- Challenges from changes in residency training, financial constraints, rapidly increasing knowledge, and limited faculty time due to increasing clinical, academic, and research demands require that new approaches are developed, including simulation, competency-based assessment, online courses and resources, and systems that reward teaching and mentorship.
- Successful mentoring is critical to the professional and personal development of students, residents, and faculty and requires significant commitment from both the mentor and the mentee.
- Coaching offers a structured approach encouraging self-reflection using facilitated feedback, analysis, and debriefing and can be individualized to each surgeon's needs and goals benefitting surgeons at all levels.
- Choosing an appropriate coach is critical, and the individual must have the knowledge and expertise to be credible coaches, strong interpersonal skills, and flexibility to adapt to each learner's different styles and needs.
- Identifying and addressing potential obstacles to coaching, including limited time, concerns about reputation, and loss of control, is important to increase "buy-in" from the learner to participate in their own performance improvement.

INTRODUCTION

Teaching and mentorship have a long history in medical education with Sir William Osler advocating for the value of learning from patients around the beginning of the twentieth century. Dr William Halsted joined Osler at Johns Hopkins and established the Halsted model for surgical training with repetitive opportunities to care for surgical patients under the supervision of a skilled surgeon, an understanding of the scientific basis of surgical diseases, and the acquisition of patient management and surgical skills with graded responsibility with each advancing year.[1] Although many surgeons have trained under this model, it is becoming increasingly clear with a national focus on patient safety, quality improvement, and continuous professional development that the current training system is inadequate. The goal of this article is to outline the specific roles and relationships that teachers, mentors, and coaches have within surgical education for the spectrum of trainees from medical students and residents through practicing surgeons (**Table 1**).

Teachers have a role in teaching a specific area of knowledge or skill and then assessing competence of their students. Teaching is generally performed over a defined period, such as a medical school rotation or residency, at the end of which students are awarded a diploma or certification.

Disclosure Statement: Both authors are surgical site mentors and proctors for Intuitive Surgical.
Section of Thoracic Surgery, University of Michigan Medical Center, 1500 E. Medical Center Drive, 2120TC/5344, Ann Arbor, MI 48109-5344, USA
* Corresponding author.
E-mail address: juleslin@umich.edu

Thorac Surg Clin 29 (2019) 311–320
https://doi.org/10.1016/j.thorsurg.2019.03.008
1547-4127/19/© 2019 Elsevier Inc. All rights reserved.

Table 1
Teachers, coaches, and mentors in thoracic surgery

	Medical Student	Resident	Fellow	Junior Faculty
Teaching	Knot tying, subcuticular suture, history and physical examinations, and patient presentations	Patient management and technical skills	Complex patient management and advanced technical skills	New techniques (robotics, minimally invasive mitral valve repair), complex patient management
Mentoring	Career paths (residency, M4 rotations), networking, scholarships, meetings to attend, research projects	Career paths, networking, research grants, meetings to attend, research projects, job openings	Career paths, networking, meetings to attend, research projects, job openings	Career paths, networking, research grants, potential collaborators, local and national committees
Coaching	Providing constructive feedback, encouragement, opportunities for practice in the operating room (OR)	Surgical techniques in OR, clinical scenarios (patient code), simulation center, mock oral examination	Surgical techniques in OR, clinical scenarios (patient code), simulation center, mock oral examination	Surgical techniques in OR, patient management, teaching techniques

Mentors can also play a role in teaching, and although teachers can also serve as mentors, mentorship tends to occur over a longer timeframe and can include guidance in areas outside of medical knowledge or surgical skills, such as career advice, networking, and work-life balance. Although teaching, mentoring, and coaching have overlapping characteristics, coaching is focused on actively identifying areas for improvement through reflecting on one's performance, making adjustments, and evaluating the impact of these changes.[2] Coaching has been widely applied and even expected in disciplines like business, music, and athletics, even for elite athletes and CEOs, but remains relatively rare in surgical education. However, with changes in surgical training with duty-hour restrictions and a greater focus on patient safety and quality improvement, changes in traditional surgical education are needed.

TEACHING

Teachers focus on specific lessons, which are usually cognitive in nature. In surgery, teaching can encompass technical skills or knowledge-based content. Lessons require instruction and formal assessment for evaluation. Because of the duration and depth of the relationship, the teacher-student relationship may not be as close as the relationship between mentors and mentees. Medical student teaching was traditionally performed during the preclinical years through lectures and frequent quizzes and examinations with rote memorization. There has been a shift toward small group sessions and increasing use of case studies, virtual and standardized patients, and suturing sessions in the simulation laboratory that are more relevant to clinical care.[3,4] With changes in medical school curricula, there has also been a push toward increasing the clinical years to give students greater clinical exposure, shifting more medical student teaching to the bedside. Changes in the curriculum are also allowing students more time for innovative electives, longitudinal patient experiences, independent study, and research, giving teachers a wider variety of opportunities to teach and mentor but also requiring more effort on the part of the student for self-directed learning. At the University of Michigan, a novel Minute Feedback System has been implemented, allowing teachers to provide timely feedback to students using a Web-based form immediately after clinic or an operative case.[5] Boot camp courses have also been developed to help medical students transition to surgical residency by practicing chest tube placement, central line placement, and tracheostomy in cadavers.[6]

Chan and colleagues[7] reported that residents felt increased confidence in transitioning to cardiothoracic residency after completing a medical student simulation course.

There have been substantial changes in cardiothoracic resident education over the last decade, and novel training approaches are needed.[8] Duty-hour restrictions have decreased the total number of hours at the bedside. Programs have adjusted by adding midlevel providers to do more routine tasks and paperwork to make those hours more educational. Residents have less continuity with their patients, and Connors and colleagues[9] found a decrease in cardiac cases logged by cardiothoracic surgery residents after duty-hour restrictions. Duty-hour restrictions have also resulted in limited exposure of general surgery trainees to cardiothoracic surgery with the elimination or fewer opportunities to rotate on the cardiac and thoracic services. There are also increasing demands on the time of teachers with increasing focus on research, clinical outcomes, and clinical revenue. With less opportunity to see complicated, less common cases, the increasing amount of medical knowledge needed, rapid advancements in technology like transcatheter techniques and robotic surgery, and less autonomy with increasing scrutiny on clinical outcomes, the simulation laboratory can be used to give residents experience managing potential intraoperative disasters, such as a massive air embolus during cardiopulmonary bypass, or opportunities to use simulators developed to train residents on various aspects of cardiac and thoracic surgery, including aortic cannulation, cardiopulmonary bypass, and robotic surgery. In addition, there are opportunities to attend an annual resident boot camp organized by the Thoracic Surgical Directors Association using high-fidelity simulators.[10,11] The American Board of Thoracic Surgery has also mandated that residents have at least 20 hours of simulation training during residency.

Technical excellence as a surgeon does not necessarily translate into excellence as a teacher. There has been an increased focus on resident education and developing more effective teachers through an Educate the Educator course for cardiothoracic surgeons.[12] Novel teaching resources, including Web-based articles, textbooks, cases, and questions curated by an editorial board of cardiothoracic surgeons, are available at learnctsurgery.sts.org to residents and surgical faculty to use for didactic sessions corresponding to the American Board of Thoracic Surgery Curriculum with a larger library of online resources at sts. webbrain.com. Although traditional textbooks are often outdated at the time of publication, electronic resources can be continuously updated and even tailored to the local curriculum. Learning management systems can also be used to track a learner's progress. An online tracheal course developed by the Joint Council on Thoracic Surgery Education was favorably received by residents, who were particularly attracted to the self-assessment quiz questions.[13]

There has been increasing recognition of adult learning theory and that adults learn better by being actively involved in their learning.[14] Knowles[14] suggested 4 principles that apply to adult learning, including the need to be involved in the planning of their instruction, experience provides the basis for learning activities, adults are most interested in subjects that are immediately relevant to their job or personal life, and adult learning is problem centered. Efforts to enable adult learners to be active participants include flipping the classroom by having residents teach interactive didactic sessions using a case-based format with a faculty moderator as opposed to a traditional lecture format. Mokadam and colleagues[15] found that flipping the classroom stimulated resident participation with residents completing both curricular readings (82%) and reviewing case presentations (79%) performing significantly better on quizzes. Similar to the Minute Feedback System, app-based feedback (Zwisch Me) has been used to provide brief, immediate written feedback to residents on their operative performance, which was most useful in addressing surgical technique and error prevention.[16] Assessment of residents is also shifting to a competency-based Milestone system rather than one based purely on time or case volume. With the expanding volume of medical knowledge and variable exposure to more complex and increasingly less common cases, competency-based assessment is needed to ensure the quality of graduating residents. The Milestones are based on specialty-specific competencies within 6 core competencies (patient care, medical knowledge, practice-based learning and improvement, professionalism, interpersonal communication skills, and systems-based practice).

To encourage teaching in the current challenging environment, new models need to be developed to recognize and reward teaching and to stimulate scholarly activity in education. Some institutions have also implemented educator tracks and education portfolios for faculty promotion. However, the requirements to advance based on these tracks vary between institutions.

MENTORING

Mentors may also be teachers, but mentoring is often more abstract and not focused on specific skill acquisition or short-term performance. According to John C. Crosby, "Mentoring is a brain to pick, an ear to listen, and a push in the right direction." Mentoring is focused on broader personal development and defining long-term goals. Mentors are often role models the mentee looks up to. Although mentorship may be a more informal process, formal mentorship programs are increasingly being used. Mentoring students and residents involves sharing advice on broader topics like career paths, networking, and work-life balance but can also provide more specific advice on selecting residency programs, research topics, or which national meetings to attend (see **Table 1**).

Mentoring styles differ but may be categorized as a Challenger, someone who pushes the mentee, asks hard questions, and helps him or her stay focused on the end goal; Cheerleader, someone who stays positive and focuses on growth; Educator, someone who takes a teaching style approach with assessments to understand the mentee's needs and then addresses any deficiencies; Ideator, someone who focuses on thinking and planning; and last, Connector, someone who helps their mentees network within their field.[17] Mentors may take on different aspects of each style, depending on the mentor's strengths and the relationship and overall goals of the mentee. A truly great mentor has the dexterity to switch between the different styles when appropriate.

Mentorship is a deeper relationship and is generally longer in duration than teaching or coaching. Whereas coaching is a more formal relationship, mentorship can be more organic and is cultivated over a longer period of time. Mentors can guide mentees in many aspects of life that are not just career related and often have similar interests or experiences as the mentee. Successful mentor-mentee relationships take commitments from both sides and can be increasingly difficult because of growing clinical, administrative, and research demands on faculty time. A study by Kibbe and colleagues[18] found that only half of departments of surgery in the United States have established mentorship programs and that most are informal and unstructured. With the importance of mentorship to career satisfaction and faculty retention, there is increasing recognition that key stakeholders need to be involved, including the department and institution. In a study by Stephens and colleagues,[19] cardiothoracic trainees' responses to questions on mentorship given with the 2017 In-Training Examination showed that although 84% had mentors, which impacted their choice of specialty in 80% of residents, and 91% viewed mentorship as critical to their success, important gaps remain, including guidance on their career path, assistance in finding a job, and advice on work-life balance.

Characteristics of a good mentor include the ability to generate enthusiasm in the mentee, the ability to inspire confidence and security, and the ability to evaluate their own effectiveness as a mentor (**Table 2**). Mentees must also fulfill their part in the relationship, including defining their goals, responsibility, follow-through, willingness to learn and improve, and timeliness. A mentoring relationship can benefit both the mentee and the mentor. Mentors not only have the satisfaction of

Table 2
Characteristics of effective teachers, mentors, and coaches

Teachers	Mentors	Coaches
Knowledgeable	Knowledgeable	Knowledgeable
Expert communication skills	Sincere	Strong interpersonal skills
Approachable	Available	Cultivates mutual trust
Passion for their subject area	Stimulates enthusiasm	Facilitates learner-directed development
Good technical skills	Trustworthy	Highly respected
Adapts to different learning styles	Flexible	Adapts approach to individual learner's goals and needs
Good listening skills	Good listening skills	Active listener
Sets clear objectives	Challenges the mentee	Recognizes the learner's abilities and experience
Strong rapport with learners	Evaluates their own effectiveness	Nonjudgmental
Organized	Track record with other mentees	

seeing the mentee succeed but also may be recognized for their efforts. Finding the right mentor can be crucial to success in any field. Physicians with successful mentorship are more likely to secure research funding, achieve promotion, have greater career satisfaction, and provide mentorship to others.[20,21] Seeking out several mentors who complement each other and different aspects of the mentee's career may also be useful with the multiple roles surgery faculty are expected to play. It is also important to recognize when a mentor is a poor match due to personality issues, lack of interest or time, or conflicts of interest and not to be afraid to change mentors.

COACHING

Although coaching includes aspects of teaching and mentoring, coaching focuses on improving and refining existing skills. There is an opportunity for coaching at all levels, and this approach can be useful throughout one's surgical career. Coaching styles can be broken down into 2 broad categories of "autonomy" and "controlling." The controlling style is the traditional, paternalistic, top-down approach to improving performance, whereas the autonomy style works to address the psychological needs of the trainee and to help develop greater self-motivation in the future.

There is significant literature on athletic coaching research to support the autonomy style in helping athletes achieve greater success compared with the controlling style. Control-style coaches provide feedback, but it is usually negative. They provide no information to their trainees on decisions and may use "punishments" to try to improve performance. The autonomy style is in direct contrast to this, and coaches learn their trainees' perspectives and understand their feelings. They provide their athletes with the information and opportunities to make their own decisions within a set of rules or limits. These coaches are approachable and avoid controlling behaviors. Athletes (and likely surgeons) who learn from autonomy-style coaches tend to develop greater intrinsic motivation and greater performance.

In medical school and residency, coaching is often done in person with a debriefing after an operative case or an event like a patient code. Debriefing involves facilitated reflection and is instrumental in the coaching process. Feedback is also crucial and emphasizes positive, good performance as well as points out areas of deficiencies and often follows debriefing as 1 fluid process. Coaching incorporates the idea of deliberate practice by actively identifying areas for improvement by reflecting on performance, making adjustments, and evaluating the impact of these changes.[2] There is increasing interest in the use of video recordings to observe technical skills and to give feedback. Videos have been used to assess and critique medical students in standardized patient interactions for many years.

In a study by Singh and colleagues,[22] medical students were randomized to receiving video-based coaching in performing laparoscopic cholecystectomy in virtual reality simulators and in the pig laboratory. Students receiving coaching outperformed control students. Bonrath and colleagues[23] reported on a randomized controlled trial comparing coaching with standard surgical training using minimally invasive Roux-en-Y gastric bypass as the index procedure. Residents in the coaching arm showed significant improvement in their technical skills and error scores. There was also improvement in self-assessment with a strong correlation between blinded video scoring and resident self-assessment in the coaching but not in the control arm with improvement in self-directed learning, skills that can benefit trainees throughout their career.

COACHING FOR SURGEONS IN PRACTICE

Although coaching has been widely applied and even expected in disciplines like business, music, and athletics, even for elite athletes and CEOs, it remains relatively rare after surgeons enter surgical practice. Surgical residency training occurs over a finite time period at the end of which surgeons are expected to be competent, and most surgeons are never observed by another surgeon after completing residency. Although surgeons often think of mastering and achieving a new skill set like transcatheter techniques or robotic surgery, they do not always consider the importance of refining that skill set with continued learning and improvement that are cornerstones of other disciplines that use coaching. Watling and colleagues[24] described a difference in learning cultures. Although surgeons emphasize mastery and competence, sports and music emphasize performance improvement. Similar to a professional athlete who can benefit from continuous feedback and refinement of their serve or golf stroke, a surgeon, who uses repetitive, technical skills, is well suited to benefit from coaching. A coach can provide an outside viewpoint that the learner cannot or does not want to see. A coach can help a surgeon change unconscious deficiencies to conscious deficiencies then to conscious abilities, and finally, to unconscious abilities.

Although it is common to think of coaching as a remedial or punitive approach, coaching should be seen as an opportunity to get constructive feedback and maximize a surgeon's potential. Coaching sessions should be nonthreatening and nonjudgmental. Finding appropriate coaches as one transitions to surgical practice is critical as well as finding lifelong mentors and coaches that help one to maintain and develop new skills after finishing traditional residency training. Coaching can be a useful approach to quality improvement, increasing a surgeon's self-awareness by identifying areas for improvement, making adjustments, and then evaluating the impact of these changes.

A structured approach using established coaching frameworks, such as PRACTICE (Problem identification, Realistic/relevant goals, Alternative solutions, Consideration of consequences, Target most feasible solutions, Implementation of Chosen solutions, and Evaluation) and GROW (Goals, Reality, Options, and Wrap-up), for laparoscopic cases can provide a systematic process that can then be personalized for individual learners based on their needs and goals.[22,25]

The Wisconsin Surgical Coaching Framework is shown in **Fig. 1**.[26] To develop a surgical coaching program, decisions should be made on whether the coaching will be live versus video based and whether this will involve expert versus peer coaching. Coaches should be identified based on their expertise and interpersonal skills. Coaches should be matched to the individual's goals and practice type and should not be direct competitors. The focus of coaching (technical, cognitive, interpersonal, and stress management) and the coaching activities (goal setting, inquiry, constructive feedback, and action planning) should also be defined.

Video-based coaching is one of the most effective methods and has been shown to be more effective than verbal feedback alone in helping to maintain behavioral changes over time.[27,28] Video allows surgeons to have a third-person view of themselves, to benchmark against other surgeons, and decreases the inaccuracy of surgeon self-assessment.[29,30] Video recording is now widely available and does not require sophisticated equipment. Videos can be reproduced and reviewed by multiple coaches. Video-based coaching also decreases many of the logistical issues and risks inherent in intraoperative teaching, including distractions from coaching that may affect concurrent patient care and ethical and medicolegal issues for coaches. Video can be fast-forwarded, making sessions more efficient and saving 50% to 80% of time without affecting the ability to assess the learner.[29,31,32] On the other hand, some operating room staff may be uncomfortable being filmed with concerns about discoverability. A gastroenterology study showed that the quality of colonoscopies improved once gastroenterologists knew they were being video recorded even if the video was not reviewed.[33] However, verbal expert review of the video is more effective than self-assessed feedback,

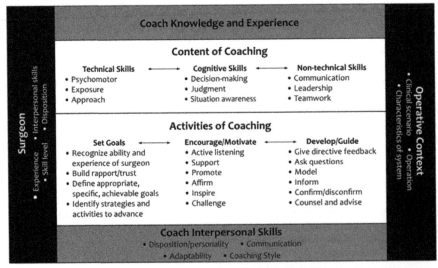

Fig. 1. Wisconsin surgical coaching framework. (*From* Greenberg CC, Ghousseini HN, Pavuluri Quamme SR, et al. Surgical coaching for individual performance improvement. Ann Surg 2015;261(1):33; with permission.)

demonstrating the added value of coaching.[34] A coaching relationship provides expertise to help identify a surgeon's gaps in knowledge or skill and to develop strategies to overcome them.[35,36]

EXPERT COACHING

There are 2 types of coaches, expert coaches and peer coaches. Expert coaching, also known as instructional coaching, involves an experienced consultant who helps a learner change their practice through self-assessment and constructive feedback. Expert coaches are especially useful when developing a new skill or procedure. Expert coaches can also provide exemplar video samples to provide good and poor examples, which can be used to help with behavior modeling of the learner. Context should be provided to the coach with a brief summary of the patient's history and presentation along with relevant radiology imaging to help put the coach in the surgeon's position. An overhead camera may also be useful to provide a complete view of the operative field with the surgeon's gross and fine movements. One example of expert coaching is the Assuring and Defining Outcomes through Procedural Training program, which uses expert coaching to teach total extraperitoneal laparoscopic hernia repair. The program included didactics, simulation training, and intraoperative training at both the coach's and the surgeon's institutions with video-based coaching for the first independent cases.[37]

PEER SURGICAL COACHING

Performance improvement for surgeons in practice, especially more senior surgeons, may be best facilitated by a peer coach. Peer coaching tends to be more bidirectional with surgeons with a similar level of experience learning from each other but can range from instructional to reciprocal approaches and should be a nonjudgmental partnership. Not all coaches are equally effective. Identifying appropriate coaches is critical, and the individuals must have the appropriate knowledge and expertise to be credible coaches (see **Table 2**). Coaches should be adaptable to each learner's different style and needs, and many of the skills needed to be an effective coach can be obtained through training. Regardless of the type of coaching, longitudinal sessions over time may help surgeons incorporate feedback into changing their performance and achieving continuous professional development.

Shubeck and colleagues[38] evaluated whether surgeons could transition to becoming a colearner for effective peer coaching. They found that participating surgeons frequently alternated between coaching and coachee roles and that the exchange of ideas was bidirectional with both surgeons offering their expertise when appropriate. One program developed in Wisconsin identified coaches using nominations through the state surgical society. Coaches underwent training sessions, and a call with participating surgeons before the coaching session was used to define goals and develop an action plan. Both coaches and participating surgeons found the coaching to be valuable.[39] According to Beasley and colleagues,[40] the framework for building effective peer coaching relationships includes aligning roles and process expectations, establishing rapport, and cultivating mutual trust.

OBSTACLES

Setting aside time for teaching, mentoring, and coaching is becoming increasingly difficult because of growing clinical, administrative, and research demands. Incorporating lessons learned through self-assessment and increased self-awareness may actually increase efficiency both inside and outside of the operating room. However, there are also other obstacles unique to coaching, including concerns about reputation and loss of control (**Table 3**). Mutabdzic and colleagues[41] performed a survey of attending surgeons evaluating perceptions of surgical coaching as a technique for performance improvement. They found that surgeons highly valued their image of competence and autonomy. Many felt threatened by surgical coaching with significant concerns about how their reputation could be affected and that even the presence of a coach could make them appear incompetent. There was also concern about feedback being given in front of colleagues.

Table 3
Barriers to surgical coaching

Concern	Approach
Limited time	Incorporating lessons learned through self-assessment and increased self-awareness may increase efficiency
Concerns about reputation	Coaching should be performed in private. Approach should be nonthreatening with the goal of improvement and not punishment
Loss of control	Individualized goals increase "buy-in" and develop self-directed learning

Surgical culture can pressure surgeons to behave a certain way to maintain an image of control and competence that makes them less likely to ask for help.[42] For coaching to be successful, it must be accepted by the surgeons involved. The learner must "buy-in" and accept the coaching process. Coaching should be performed in a private setting and can be done away from patients and colleagues using a video-based approach.[31] However, the need to maintain one's image must be balanced with the value of receiving immediate feedback before the teaching points are forgotten. These issues may need to be negotiated to establish trust between the coach and the learner, and feedback should be tailored to each surgeon's learning styles and needs. The approach should be nonthreatening with the goal of improvement and not punishment.

Many surgeons do not feel the need for coaching and fear the loss of control. However, there are several studies showing that physician self-assessment is inaccurate and that surgeons would benefit from external coaching.[43–45] Creating individualized goals, defined by the learner, helps to increase "buy-in" and to develop self-directed learning, which can improve the surgeon's sense of control over their own performance improvement. The coaching relationship is a partnership, and the coach is helping the learner help themselves.

FUTURE

As technology continues to improve, remote video review and coaching by teleconference may become more common, improving efficiency and even anonymity, which remains an obstacle for some seeking out coaching opportunities. Video conferencing may be particularly useful for surgeons practicing in remote areas or in solo practice, where there is a lack of experienced partners and access to traditional learning opportunities. Technology is also being developed for surgical telementoring with important criteria, including safety, reliability, transmission quality, ease of use, and cost.[46]

As coaching becomes more common, it will be important to create training opportunities for coaches to both learn and share a wide range of coaching techniques and strategies. Regional and national surgical societies and quality collaboratives can play an important role in identifying expert and peer coaches, training programs, and networks to distribute ideas and resources. More research will also need to be done to confirm that coaching results in better patient outcomes.

SUMMARY

Teaching, mentoring, and coaching all play critical roles in success at all levels from medical students to cardiothoracic residents and faculty. However, challenges due to changes in residency training, regulatory and financial constraints, rapidly increasing knowledge and technology, and limited faculty time due to increasing clinical, academic, and research demands require that new approaches are developed using simulation, competency-based assessment, online courses and resources, and the development of systems that reward teaching and mentorship and encourage scholarly activity in education. Although coaching has been used effectively in other disciplines, including athletics, business, and music, surgical coaching remains relatively uncommon. However, there is growing interest due to an increasing focus on safety and quality improvement and the realization that current continuing medical education is limited. Coaching offers a structured approach encouraging self-reflection using facilitated feedback, analysis, and debriefing and can be individualized to each surgeon's needs and goals and can benefit surgeons at all levels.

REFERENCES

1. Grillo HC. To impart this art: the development of graduate surgical education in the United States. Surgery 1999;125(1):1–14.
2. Ericsson KA. Deliberate practice and the acquisition and maintenance of expert performance in medicine and related domains. Acad Med 2004;79(10 Suppl): S70–81.
3. Cendan J, Lok B. The use of virtual patients in medical school curricula. Adv Physiol Educ 2012;36(1):48–53.
4. Anderson MB, Stillman PL, Wang Y. Growing use of standardized patients in teaching and evaluation in medical education. Teach Learn Med 1994;6(1): 15–22.
5. Hughes DT, Leininger L, Reddy RM, et al. A novel minute feedback system for medical students. Am J Surg 2017;213(2):330–5.
6. Tocco N, Brunsvold M, Kabbani L, et al. Innovation in internship preparation: an operative anatomy course increases senior medical students' knowledge and confidence. Am J Surg 2013;206(2):269–79.
7. Chan PG, Schaheen LW, Chan EG, et al. Technology-enhanced simulation improves trainee readiness transitioning to cardiothoracic training. J Surg Educ 2018;75(5):1395–402.
8. Vaporciyan AA, Yang SC, Baker CJ, et al. Cardiothoracic surgery residency training: past, present, and future. J Thorac Cardiovasc Surg 2013;146(4):759–67.

9. Connors RC, Doty JR, Bull DA, et al. Effect of work-hour restriction on operative experience in cardiothoracic surgical residency training. J Thorac Cardiovasc Surg 2009;137(3):710–3.

10. Hicks GL, Gangemi J, Angona RE, et al. Cardiopulmonary bypass simulation at the Boot Camp. J Thorac Cardiovasc Surg 2011;141(1):284–92.

11. Fann JI, Feins RH, Hicks GL, et al. Evaluation of simulation training in cardiothoracic surgery: the senior tour perspective. J Thorac Cardiovasc Surg 2012;143(2):264–72.

12. Yang SC, Vaporciyan AA, Mark RJ, et al. The Joint Council on Thoracic Surgery Education (JCTSE) "educate the educators" faculty development course: analysis of the first 5 Years. Ann Thorac Surg 2016;102(6):2127–32.

13. Antonoff MB, Verrier ED, Yang CC, et al. Online learning in thoracic surgical training: promising results of multi-institutional pilot study. Ann Thorac Surg 2014;98(3):1057–63.

14. Knowles M. The adult learner: a neglected species. 3rd edition. Houston (TX): Gulf Publishing; 1984.

15. Mokadam NA, Dardas TF, Hermsen JL, et al. Flipping the classroom: case-based learning, accountability, assessment, and feedback leads to a favorable change in culture. J Thorac Cardiovasc Surg 2017;153(4):987–96.e1.

16. Karim AS, Sternbach JM, Bender EM, et al. Quality of operative performance feedback given to thoracic surgery residents using an app-based system. J Surg Educ 2017;74(6):981–7.

17. Hughes A. The 5 best types of mentors. New York: Huffington Post; 2013. Available at: https://www.huffingtonpost.com/anthony-hughes/the-5-best-types-of-mentors_b_4149657.html. Accessed January 19, 2019.

18. Kibbe MR, Pellegrini CA, Townsend CM, et al. Characterization of mentorship programs in departments of surgery in the United States. JAMA Surg 2016;151(10):900–6.

19. Stephens EH, Goldstone AB, Fiedler AG, et al. Appraisal of mentorship in cardiothoracic surgery training. J Thorac Cardiovasc Surg 2018;156(6):2216–23.

20. Palepu A, Friedman RH, Barnett RC, et al. Junior faculty members' mentoring relationships and their professional development in U.S. medical schools. Acad Med 1998;73(3):318–23.

21. Benson CA, Morahan PS, Sachdeva AK, et al. Effective faculty preceptoring and mentoring during reorganization of an academic medical center. Med Teach 2002;24(5):550–7.

22. Singh P, Aggarwal R, Tahir M, et al. A randomized controlled study to evaluate the role of video-based coaching in training laparoscopic skills. Ann Surg 2015;261(5):862–9.

23. Bonrath EM, Dedy NJ, Gordon LE, et al. Comprehensive surgical coaching enhances surgical skill in the operating room: a randomized controlled trial. Ann Surg 2015;262(2):205–12.

24. Watling C, Driessen E, van der Vleuten CPM, et al. Music lessons: revealing medicine's learning culture through a comparison with that of music. Med Educ 2013;47(8):842–50.

25. Palmer S. PRACTICE: a model suitable for coaching, counselling, psychotherapy and stress management. Coaching Psychologist 2007;3(2):71–7.

26. Greenberg CC, Ghousseini HN, Pavuluri Quamme SR, et al. Surgical coaching for individual performance improvement. Ann Surg 2015;261(1):32–4.

27. Scherer LA, Chang MC, Meredith JW, et al. Videotape review leads to rapid and sustained learning. Am J Surg 2003;185(6):516–20.

28. Birnbach DJ, Santos AC, Bourlier RA, et al. The effectiveness of video technology as an adjunct to teach and evaluate epidural anesthesia performance skills. Anesthesiology 2002;96(1):5–9.

29. Ward M, MacRae H, Schlachta C, et al. Resident self-assessment of operative performance. Am J Surg 2003;185(6):521–4.

30. Martin D, Regehr G, Hodges B, et al. Using videotaped benchmarks to improve the self-assessment ability of family practice residents. Acad Med 1998;73(11):1201–6.

31. Dath D, Regehr G, Birch D, et al. Toward reliable operative assessment: the reliability and feasibility of videotaped assessment of laparoscopic technical skills. Surg Endosc 2004;18(12):1800–4.

32. Beard JD, Jolly BC, Newble DI, et al. Assessing the technical skills of surgical trainees. Br J Surg 2005;92(6):778–82.

33. Rex DK, Hewett DG, Raghavendra M, et al. The impact of videorecording on the quality of colonoscopy performance: a pilot study. Am J Gastroenterol 2010;105(11):2312–7.

34. Porte MC, Xeroulis G, Reznick RK, et al. Verbal feedback from an expert is more effective than self-accessed feedback about motion efficiency in learning new surgical skills. Am J Surg 2007;193(1):105–10.

35. Gagliardi AR, Wright FC. Exploratory evaluation of surgical skills mentorship program design and outcomes. J Contin Educ Health Prof 2010;30(1):51–6.

36. Marguet CG, Young MD, L'Esperance JO, et al. Hand assisted laparoscopic training for postgraduate urologists: the role of mentoring. J Urol 2004;172(1):286–9.

37. Greenberg JA, Jolles S, Sullivan S, et al. A structured, extended training program to facilitate adoption of new techniques for practicing surgeons. Surg Endosc 2018;32(1):217–24.

38. Shubeck SP, Kanters AE, Sandhu G, et al. Dynamics within peer-to-peer surgical coaching relationships: early evidence from the Michigan Bariatric Surgical Collaborative. Surgery 2018;164(2):185–8.

39. Greenberg CC, Ghousseini HN, Pavuluri Quamme SR, et al. A statewide surgical coaching program provides opportunity for continuous professional development. Ann Surg 2018;267(5): 868–73.

40. Beasley HL, Ghousseini HN, Wiegmann DA, et al. Strategies for building peer surgical coaching relationships. JAMA Surg 2017;152(4):e165540.

41. Mutabdzic D, Mylopoulos M, Murnaghan ML, et al. Coaching surgeons: is culture limiting our ability to improve? Ann Surg 2015;262(2):213–6.

42. Jin CJ, Martimianakis MA, Kitto S, et al. Pressures to "measure up" in surgery: managing your image and managing your patient. Ann Surg 2012;256(6): 989–93.

43. Regehr G, Mylopoulos M. Maintaining competence in the field: learning about practice, through practice, in practice. J Contin Educ Health Prof 2008; 28(Suppl 1):S19–23.

44. Brydges R, Dubrowski A, Regehr G. A new concept of unsupervised learning: directed self-guided learning in the health professions. Acad Med 2010; 85(10 Suppl):S49–55.

45. Davis DA, Mazmanian PE, Fordis M, et al. Accuracy of physician self-assessment compared with observed measures of competence: a systematic review. JAMA 2006;296(9):1094–102.

46. Erridge S, Yeung DKT, Patel HRH, et al. Telementoring of surgeons: a systematic review. Surg Innov 2018. https://doi.org/10.1177/1553350618813250.

Faculty Development
Using Education for Career Advancement

Gregory D. Rushing, MD, Nahush A. Mokadam, MD*

KEYWORDS

- Academic surgery • Surgical education • Promotion and tenure • Clinical educator

KEY POINTS

- The Clinical Educator track appropriately rewards effort for those involved in Surgical Education with regard to promotion and tenure.
- Clinical Education is not just teaching: educational scholarship requires assessment of learning, efficiency of teaching techniques, curriculum development, and evolution.
- Institutional and academic advancement requires development of skills, measurement of progress, obtaining funding, and professional presentation of project outcomes.

INTRODUCTION

Academic advancement has transformed in the last decade. There are now multiple "pathways" forward in academic promotion and tenure. Faculty development occurs throughout the promotion and tenure process but is thought to be most formative early on, at the start of an academic career. Effective advancement from assistant to associate to full professor requires (1) defined short- and long-term goals and (2) understanding institutional definition and measurement of success.

Historically, academic surgeons developed a specialized clinical practice, oversaw a benchtop research laboratory, and taught residents as well as medical students. This was the so-called "triple threat" approach to career advancement. Measurable success in clinical practice and grantsmanship was essential, while education was implicit in the role. This required a large portion of time in clinical practice, performing research, speaking at conferences, publishing manuscripts, and obtaining independent funding. Research and publication are rewarded at uneven rates over education.[1] Because professional fee for service has been reduced, along with the increased scrutiny on clinical "presence" and research commitment, the ability to maintain simultaneous excellence in both clinical and investigative efforts has become increasingly rare.[2–4] The ability for a full-time clinical surgeon to compete for National Institutes of Health dollars is challenging and, in many cases, impossible. Further, a more informed public, outcome tracking/publishing, and star ratings have led to a more "hands on" approach to clinical endeavors, even in academic surgery. All the while, the unfunded mandate of education remains in the shadows. Still today, the 3 legs of the academic mission are not equal.

In the last decade, however, many academic institutions have developed alternate and nontraditional "tracks" to promote and reward the effort that is required in an educational program.

Disclosure Statement: G.D. Rushing is an investigator for Abbott and Medtronic. N.A. Mokadam is an investigator and consultant for Abbott, Medtronic, and SynCardia.
Division of Cardiac Surgery, Department of Surgery, The Ohio State University Wexner Medical Center, Columbus, OH, USA
* Corresponding author. Division of Cardiac Surgery, N-825 Doan Hall, 410 West 10th Avenue, Columbus, OH 43210.
E-mail address: Nahush.Mokadam@osumc.edu

Educators have both embraced and suffered from this distinction. On one hand, these alternate tracks have allowed for appropriate promotion and tenure in the highest academic centers.[5] Unfortunately, in some settings, this has also led to the development of a dual, or multicaste system in which the "Educator" track is (un)consciously devalued. The fault in this system is somewhat our own as outlined later.

DEVELOPING SKILLS

The foundation of being a clinical educator is teaching. Most surgical faculty are required to do some level of teaching, whether in the operating room, on the wards, or in the outpatient setting. This requires being an excellent clinician. Becoming an expert surgeon with solid clinical acumen and outcomes is paramount to respect and advancement in the department and institution. Lectures to residents and students are also routinely given. Simple instruction, lectures, or teaching of medical students and residents is not enough to be defined as a clinical educator, because all academic surgeons do this. Unfortunately, many have rested their laurels on these processes. Formal education training was not sought, and educational efficacy was not measured.

During the training of a doctor and surgeon, very little, if any, emphasis is given to the quality of teaching. For faculty using education as their academic focus, this is an enormous opportunity for improvement. Assessment of learning and efficacy of teaching techniques is imperative to appropriate curriculum development and evolution. Many options are available for young faculty to improve their teaching skills.[6] The American College of Surgeons (ACS) has a week-long intensive course organized annually called the Surgeons as Educators Course. It is focused on 4 topics: (1) teaching skills, (2) curriculum development, (3) administration and leadership, and (4) performance and program development.[7] Techniques focus on adult learning models and fostering and effective learning environment, especially with the specific and unique needs of medical students and residents. Development of clerkship and residency rotations with validated assessment tools are mapped out. Administrative responsibility such as motivating faculty, implementing change, and conflict resolution are discussed. Because of the popularity of the ACS program and waiting lists, the Joint Council on Thoracic Surgery Education, Inc. developed a similar course specific for cardiothoracic surgery named "Educate the Educator."[8] Although this course was active,

sessions taught each year in this 3-day course included the following:

- Assessment of Surgical Skills
- Cashing-in on Your Educational Portfolio
- Converting Educational Effort into Promotional Currency
- Curriculum Design
- Formative Feedback
- How People Learn
- Teaching in the Operating Room
- Teaching Psychomotor Skills

The Stanford Faculty Development Center for Medical Teachers offers training to medical school and academic health center faculty to develop and conduct teaching courses at their home institutions.[9] Effectively, "teaching others to teach" course includes (1) learning climate, (2) communication of goals, (3) understanding and retention, (4) evaluation, and (5) feedback and self-directed learning. There are also workshops to benefit those teaching basic science as well.

The annual meetings of the Association for Surgical Education (ASE) as well as the ACS offer multiple opportunities for advanced teaching skills. In addition, the ASE offers annual courses to clerkship directors and coordinators on how to run a surgical clerkship. The Association of Academic Surgeons' "The Fundamentals of Surgical Research" course has sections on educational research. The Association of Program Directors in Surgery offers a course to all new program directors. When embarking on becoming a clinical educator, negotiate to attend one or more of these resources while accepting leadership positions and administrative appointments such as clerkship or program directors.

In order to advance in surgical education, using these types of programs can help establish credibility to students and colleagues, as well as the Promotion and Tenure committees. Not only does this demonstrate commitment and focus but also provides valuable skills to the developing faculty member. In addition, just like with clinical skills, the need for lifelong learning in educational science is important. Participation in national meetings and educational fora further validate education as a means for career development.

MEASURING PROGRESS: THE TEACHING PORTFOLIO

The teaching portfolio has been well described and is a mandatory component of the clinical educator's pathway to promotion and is a good way to ensure all types of teaching activity are recognized.[10] Teaching portfolios are increasingly used for promotion consideration irrespective of a pathway in many centers. The teaching portfolio gives thorough and consistent documentation of a faculty member's educational activities and is a companion to the more traditional curriculum vitae. Organization of a teaching portfolio varies from center to center and represents the following general categories:

Reflective Statement

The reflective statement should be a one-page essay on teaching philosophy, and this may include short- and long-term goals, strategies for improvement of teaching, areas of research interest, and your personal motivation for teaching.

Introductory Statement

The introductory statement defines the educator's role as related to teaching responsibilities, percentage of effort, courses taught, and area of research. This may include titles (ie, Program Director, Clerkship Director) that are both formal and informal. Specific scholarly activities should be highlighted.

Direct Teaching Activities

The direct teaching activities section should list all teaching efforts, curriculum and materials development, learner assessments, creation of enduring educational materials, educational administration and leadership activities, evidence of mentoring, and professional development in education. Giving lectures to medical undergraduates is generally well documented, because it is often recorded and reported easily; however, resident lectures, journal clubs, wet laboratories, and community continuing medical education (CME) activities are often unreported. Curriculum development, however minor it might seem, is also a hallmark of an effective educator.

Appendix

The appendix compiles copies of teaching awards, certificates, degrees, and honors received.

There are software and web-based programs to track activities and help assemble a portfolio. Often institutions have required tools that are mandated for use. The teaching portfolio is best compiled and updated on a regular basis and not left to a subordinate or administrative assistant. The often-unreported effort of the clinical educator is due to the inability to remember specific educational activities.

FORMALIZING EDUCATION

Participation in the organization of medical education is an important aspect of career development for the clinical educator. Opportunities in organized medical education include the undergraduate medical admission committees, academic review committees, and positions of Clerkship Director for medical students and Program Director for residents. Assistant level positions for these roles provide initial administrative experience in formal education and should be sought. Participation (as faculty) in local, regional, and national courses and CME events can expand formal educational experience. These experiences at your home institution can lead to leadership positions in various regional and national organizations, specifically those promoting surgical clinical education (**Box 1**). Local and regional organizations are often more accommodating of junior faculty, leading to more experience and better performance at the national level.

The Promotion and Tenure Committee at most institutions requires regional reputation for promotion to Associate Professor and national reputation for attaining Full Professor rank. It is therefore imperative for participation in formal processes, courses, and societies to achieve these milestones.

Box 1 Organizations for surgical education resources	
American College of Surgeons	http://www.facs.org/education
Association for Surgical Education	http://www.surgicaleducation.com
Association for Academic Surgery	http://www.aasurg.org
Association of Program Directors in Surgery	http://www.apds.org
Society of University Surgeons	http://www.susweb.org
Society of Thoracic Surgeons	http://www.sts.org
Thoracic Surgery Directors Association	http://www.tsda.org

EDUCATIONAL SCHOLARSHIP

Educational scholarship, like any innovative research, requires creativity, planning, and, ultimately, execution. Whereas a basic scientist would carefully design an experiment, gather reagents, perform analyses, and interpret the results for publication, the same fundamental principles remain in place in the field of education. Clinical educators usually maintain busy clinical practices, provide quality education to their trainees, and must be cognizant of opportunities, because they are generally widely available. Examples of such opportunities include curriculum development (including validation), novel assessment tools, and innovative practice efficiencies, among many others. Transforming these processes into a research project and subsequently completing the analysis for peer-reviewed publication can be as equally challenging as gel electrophoresis. Educational scholarship is presented at multiple national meetings (Association for Surgical Education, Association for Academic Surgery, American College of Surgeons) and their associated journals publish education-related manuscripts; it is also increasingly a part of specialty specific meetings (Society of Thoracic surgeons [STS], American Association for Thoracic Surgery [AATS]).

The ASE offers a Surgical Education Research Fellowship.[11] This is a 1-year stay-at-home fellowship designed to equip the surgeon with skills needed to perform and succeed at research in surgical education. It begins at the ASE annual meeting where the fellow is provided the basics needed to conduct, apply, and publish educational research. Then each participant is matched carefully with a mentor and develops a project for development. In the fall, progress is reported at the American College of Surgeons Clinical Congress. This program specifically focuses on how to research the literature, design a project with appropriate methodologies, and translate that project into published presentations.

The Association of American Medical Colleges has a certificate program available through their Group on Educational Affairs: the Medical Education Research Certificate.[12] The program is designed for clinicians, who have little experience with medical education research, to understand the purpose, process, and become effective collaborators. These programmatic workshops are dedicated to specific education research areas and can be taken in any order:

- Data Management and Preparing for Statistical Consultation
- Formulating Research Questions and Designing Studies

- Hypothesis-Driven Research
- Measuring Educational Outcomes with Reliability and Validity
- Introduction to Qualitative Data Collection Methods
- Program Evaluation and Evaluation Research
- Qualitative Analysis Methods in Medical Education
- Questionnaire Design and Survey Research
- Searching and Evaluating the Medical Education Literature
- Scholarly Writing: Publishing Medical Education Research

The Harvard Macy Institute is a collaborative effort that offers 3 different programs to provide advanced training to leaders in health education.[13] Each of these 3 programs offers something different for clinical educators throughout their career paths. *The Program for Educators in Health Professions* is designed for physicians, scientists, and other health care professionals who are educators; its specific goal is to enhance professional development in learning and teaching, curriculum, evaluation, leadership, and information technology. *The Systems Approach to Assessment in Health Professions Education* is designed to address learning and assessment of competencies, teaching, and program efficacy. Each participant learns to refine the assessment and evaluation challenges specific to their institution. The *Leading Innovations in Heath Care and Education Program* is directed at education leaders. Its specific goal is to enable these leaders to develop and implement their own "action plans" to fulfill their institution's educational mission.

FUNDING FOR RESEARCH

Approximately two-thirds of published medical education studies are not funded, and those studies remain significantly underfunded when you measure specific "percentage effort" performed by each investigator.[14] Many national professional organizations, charitable organizations, state, and institutional sources fund research but are limited to specific proposals of interest to them. Notably, our national societies in Thoracic Surgery (STS, AATS, Western Thoracic Surgery Association, The Southern Thoracic Surgical Association) all have educational awards and foundations (Thoracic Surgery Foundation, Graham Foundation), which have a peer-reviewed process to support scholarly activity in education. Larger organizations (American Heart Association, American College of Cardiology) have nationally competitive educational grants and frequently seek surgical projects. In addition, pilot research projects funded from within a hospital or department may be available. Mentorship from within or from a nationally recognized educator may help identify appropriate sources of funding.

Finding the most appropriate funding source and reviewing submission requirements are key starting points. Examination of the agency's prior funded projects and review of the objectives can guide the best submissions. As with any grant, careful assessment of personal strengths and weaknesses, available institutional resources and support, potential collaborations, and time commitment/restraints are required. Development of a realistic timeline is important in order to manage expectations: 1 year to obtain preliminary data, 1 to 2 months for Institutional Review Board and Institutional Animal Care and Use Committee approval, 1 to 2 months for grant writing, and about 9 months from grant submission through review and to funding. Deadlines are strict and generally nonnegotiable for a given funding cycle.

There are several search engines that will permit search irrespective of specialty or special interest (**Box 2**). These include the Community of Science, which is likely the most comprehensive source of funding for research on the web. Grants.gov is the single point of access for more than 900 grant programs provided by the federal grant-making agencies, 26 of them in total. Health and Humans Services specific grant information can be found at GrantsNet, where more than 300 programs are listed. The "Foundation Center and "Pivot" provides news and information and maintain databases of active grants and grant makers.

Several sources exist specifically for surgical education (**Box 3**). The Center for Excellence in Surgical Education, Research, and Training grant (up to $25,000) is provided by the foundation arm of the ASE.[15] These grants provide funds to advance surgical education research. The ASE lists several priorities, which include Innovations in Performance Evaluation and Assessment, Innovations in Medical Student Programs, Innovations in Resident and Faculty Development, and

Innovations in Educational Administration. The Roslyn Faculty Research award from the AAS provides early career support ($35,000) for young faculty members in direct cost incurred during the conduct of proposed research.[16] Although not specific to educational research, it is not limited. In this case, early career is defined as less than 5 years from completion of residency and not having attained the rank of Associate Professor. The AAS also provides a Research Fellowship Award ($20,000) to eligible residents or fellows involved in clinical outcome, health services, or education research.[11] The resident is paired with an AAS member. Applicants must have completed 2 years of a surgical residency, and the award may go toward salary support. The Society of University Surgeons also provides awards for resident and early faculty ($00,000). The grants are intended for trainees or faculty within their first 3 years from residency completion, who are performing research focused on surgical innovation, bioengineering, or surgical education.[17,18] The ACS Resident Research Scholarship offers 2-year ($30,000 each) support for residents in a surgical or surgical specialty program who has completed 2 years of postdoctoral training. The funds support research but not salary.[19]

Other sources not specific to surgery are specific to educational research (**Box 4**). The American Educational Research Association, supported by the National Science Foundation, awards projects that quantitatively evaluate data that have US education policy relevance.[20] The Agency for Healthcare Research and Quality provides funds that are aimed to improve patient safety.[21] Recently, simulation and education research has been an interest to the agency.[4,22] The Stemmler Medical Education Research Fund is provided by the National Board of Medical Examiners for research projects in assessment and evaluation.[23] Small educational research projects can be funded ($5000 or $7500) by the Southern Group on Educational Affairs (a subgroup of the Association of American Medical Colleges).[24] These are designed to be start-up funds and

---

Box 2
Search engines and federal funding sources

Community of Science	http://www.cos.com
Grants.gov	http://www.grants.gov
Health and Human Services	http://www.hhs.gov/grantsnet/
The Foundation Center	http://www.foundationcenter.org
Ex Libris Pivot	http://www.exlibrisgroup.com/products/pivot
National Institutes of Health	http://www.grants.nih.gov
Health Resources and Services Administration	http://www.hrsa.gov/grants
National Science Foundation	http://www.nsf.gov

Box 3
Surgical specific funding sources

ASE CESERT Program	http://www.surgicaleducation.com/cesert-grants
AAS Roslyn Faculty Research Award	http://www.aasurg.org/awards/roslyn-faculty-award/
AAS Research Fellowship Award	http://www.aasurg.org/awards/fellowship-award
SUS Junior Faculty Award	http://www.susweb.org/junior-faculty-award
SUS Resident Scholar Award	http://www.susweb.org/sus-resident-scholar-award
ACS Resident Research Scholarship	http://www.facs.org/memberservices/acsresident.html

---

seek to stimulate further activity. Special promotion is given to collaborative projects across institutions.

Funding for medical education is limited, but opportunities for the clinical educator are present. Applicant persistence, like for all grants, is the key to success. Skills needed for successful planning, methodology, and grantsmanship may be enhanced by pursuing an advanced degree in medical education.

ADVANCED DEGREES

Pursuit of a formal degree for those interested in dedicating their time and career to surgical education may be advisable. Exposure to educational philosophy and teaching methodology make one a more effective educator, which then can be used in daily teaching of medical students and residents. Coursework in curriculum development and curriculum assessment are useful for those interested in becoming medical student clerkship and residency program directors. Exposure to educational policy and administration, along with educational infrastructure and leadership, are beneficial in the rise to the ranks of departmental Vice Chair of Surgical Education or even Dean.

The traditional model of committing at least 2 years of research during surgical residency training does not prepare the surgical clinical educator for health services or education research. The use of quantitative as well as qualitative research methods, a skill set not easily learned outside of a classroom, is difficult in the traditional surgical residency model. Research in

education often deals with variables that are difficult to control, and learning is notoriously difficult to assess quantitatively or qualitatively. Accepted methodologies such as pre- and posttesting, surveys, interviews, and observation are often learned in advanced degree programs. Of all the degrees that can be applied to research in surgical education, the traditional master's degree or Doctorate of Philosophy in Education (PhD) is the most broad, extensive, and likely beneficial.

Not including the financial implications of obtaining an advanced degree is the significant time commitment, which is often more difficult when combined with the length of cardiothoracic surgical training. A master's degree in education may be obtained in 1 year, but the PhD will usually require a minimum of 3 years. Courses focus on qualitative and quantitative research methods as well as curriculum development and assessment that are widely applicable to surgical educators. Many graduate school education programs have a significant portion of their curriculum devoted to child and adolescent education, not necessarily useful for adult educators, and should therefore be carefully evaluated in order to avoid focus on less relevant material.

Given the distinct needs of medical education, there are several graduate degree programs that have been specifically developed for health care professionals. The master's degree in Education for the Health Professions and the master's degree of Health Profession Education are specifically designed to fill these needs. The master's in Public Health or master's in Clinical Investigation or Clinical Epidemiology have a strong focus on quantitative research methods and can certainly

---

Box 4
Educational specific funding sources

AERA	http://www.aera.net
AHRQ	http://www.ahrq.gov.fund
Stemmler Medical Education Fund	http://www.nbme.org/research/stemmler
SGEA (AAMC)	http://aamc.org/members/gea/regions/sgea/awards
Society of University Surgeons	http://www.susweb.org
Society of Thoracic Surgeons	http://www.sts.org
Thoracic Surgery Directors Association	http://www.tsda.org

be helpful for a career focusing on education research. More than 30 programs across the country specific to health professional education are described on the ASE Website.[25] Specific surgical education programs are also available. The Imperial College of London[26] and the University of Dundee in Scotland[27] provide advanced degrees with the specific goal in mind of producing future leaders in surgical education. The University of Dundee program, endorsed by the Royal College of Surgeons of Edinburgh, is a complete virtual online learning environment using peer and tutor interaction: via blogs, podcasts, discussion boards, webinar, and video clips. The number of institutions using online and virtual environments may help with time management for the surgeon who also needs to maintain a clinical practice.

SUMMARY

The clinical educator is one of several pathways or tracks that can be followed for promotion and advancement. Faculty development in surgical education has specific and inherently different challenges from the traditional academic tenure track. Surgical clinical education is more than just teaching: curriculum development, assessment, validation, and innovative practice efficiencies are necessary skills that must be cultivated. Turning these into successful projects that are presented and published is crucial for success and promotion, and this can be accomplished by developing skills, measuring progress, and obtaining funding and advanced degrees. Mentorship and exposure are key for faculty development in the area of education.

REFERENCES

1. Thomas PA, Diener-West M, Canto MI, et al. Results of an academic promotion and career path survey of faculty at the Johns Hopkins Univerity School of Medicine. Acad Med 2004;79:258–64.
2. McCook A. Duke fraud case highlights financial risks for universities. Science 2016;353:977–8.
3. Bauchner H, Fontanarosa P, Flanagin A, et al. Scientific misconduct and medical journals. JAMA 2018; 320:1985–7.
4. Feins RH, Burkhart HM, Conte JV, et al. Simulation-based training in cardiac surgery. Ann Thorac Surg 2017;103:312–21.
5. The Ohio State University College of Medicine. The Ohio State University College of Medicine faculty advancement, mentoring and engagement (FAME) 2016. Available at: https://medicine.osu.edu/faculty/fame/Pages/index.aspx. Accessed November 20, 2018.
6. Sanfey H, Gantt NL. Career development resource: academic career in surgical education. Am J Surg 2012;204:126–9.
7. American College of Surgeons. Introdiction to Surgeons as Educators. 2018. Available at: http://www.facs.org/education/sre/aseintro.html. Accessed November 22, 2018.
8. Yang SC, Vaporciyan AA, Mark RJ, et al. The Joint Council on Thoracic Surgery Education (JCTSE) "Educate the educators" faculty development course: analysis of the first 5 years. Ann Thorac Surg 2016;102:2127–32.
9. Stanford School of Medicine. Stanford Faculty Devlopment Center for Medical Teachers. 2016. Available at: http://www.sfdc.stanford.edu. Accessed November 22, 2018.
10. Univeristy of Virginia, School of Medicine. UVa SOM teaching portfolio. Charlottesville (VA); University of Virginia School of Medicine Facutly Affairs and Development; 2018. Available at: https://faculty.med.virginia.edu/facultyaffairs/teaching-portfolio/. Accessed November 20, 2018.
11. Association for Surgical Education. Surgical education research fellowship 2017. Available at: http://surgicaleducation.com/surgical-education-research-fellowship-overview/. Accessed November 22, 2018.
12. AAMC. Asociation of Medical Colleges Professional Development. Medical Education Research Certificate Program. Available at: http://aamc.org/members/gea/merc/. Accessed November 19, 2018.
13. Harvard Macy Institute. 2017. Available at: http://www.harvardmacy.org. Accessed November 20, 2018.
14. Reed DA, Kern DE, Levine RB, et al. Costs and funding for published medical education research. JAMA 2005;294:1052–7.
15. The Association for Surgical Education. CESERT grants program. Available at: http://www.surgicaleducation.com/cesert-grants. Accessed November 23, 2018.
16. Association for Academic Surgery. Joel J. Roslyn Faculty Research Award. Available at: http://www.aasurg.org/awards/roslyn-faculty-award/. Accessed November 23, 2018.
17. Society of University Surgeons. Resident research scholar award. Available at: https://www.susweb.org/resident-scholar-research-awards/. Accessed November 23, 2018.
18. Society of University Surgeons. Junior faculty research award 2016. Available at: https://www.susweb.org/junior-faculty-award/. Accessed November 23, 2018.
19. American College of Surgeons. ACS Resident Research Scholarship. Available at: http://www.facs.org/member-services/scholarship/resident/acsresident. Accessed November 24, 2018.

20. American Educational Research Association. Professional Opportunities Funding. AERA Grants Program. Available at: http://www.aera.net/ProfessionalOpportunitiesFunding/FundingOpportunities/AERAGrantsProgram/ResearchGrants. Accessed November 24, 2018.

21. Agency for Healthcare Research and Quality. Funding and Grants. Available at: http://www.ahrq.gov/funding. Accessed November 24, 2018.

22. Mokadam NA, Fann JI, Hicks GL, et al. Experience with the cardiac surgery simulation curriculum: results of the resident and faculty survey. Ann Thorac Surg 2017;103:322–8.

23. National Board of Medical Examiners. Edward J. Stemmler Medical Education Research fund. Available at: http://www.nbme.org/research/stemmler.html. Accessed November 24, 2018.

24. Association of American Medical Colleges. Medical Education Research Grants. Southern Group on Educational Affairs. Available at: http://www.aamc.org/members/gea/regions/sgea/awards/66884/sgea_research.html. Accessed November 24, 2018.

25. The Association for Surgical Education. The Association for Surgical Education Advanced Degrees. Available at: http://surgicaleducation.com/view/advanced-degrees/. Accessed November 22, 2018.

26. Imperial College of London. Imperial College of London Surgical Education. Available at: http://www.imperial.ac.uk/study/pg/medicine/surgical-education/. Accessed November 23, 2018.

27. University of Dundee. Post-Graduate Education. PGCert Medical Education (for Surgeons). Available at: https://www.dundee.ac.uk/study/pg/med-ed-surgeons. Accessed November 19, 2018.

Virtual or Augmented Reality to Enhance Surgical Education and Surgical Planning

Christopher Cao, MBBS, BSc, PhD, FRACS[a],
Robert J. Cerfolio, MD, MBA, FCCP[b],*

KEYWORDS

- Augmented reality • Computed tomography • MRI • Virtual reality

KEY POINTS

- Virtual reality and augmented reality technologies have an increasing presence in surgical practice.
- Existing evidence demonstrates improvement in both clinical outcomes and surgical training.
- Standardized, quantitative measurements and evolving technology will likely increase utilization of AR and VR technologies in the health sector.

There has been an exponential growth in the development and interest in virtual reality (VR) and augmented reality (AR) including in the medical field as shown in **Fig. 1**. VR is a form of computer-generated technology that combines a multifaceted virtual environment to create a realistic multisensory imagery for the observer to feel a presence in another world.[1] The observer can interact with the virtual environment, including haptic systems that can provide tactile feedback and mechanical sensations.[1] On the other hand, AR overlays generated data over a real or live image, in order to modify, superimpose, or enrich the actual live image.[2] VR can be thought of as a replacement of reality with a virtual environment, whereas AR enhances certain elements of the real world with additional overlaying data. This review provides an overview of the current applications of AR and VR in surgical education and surgical planning and explores the future directions and challenges in this expanding field.

There is a wide range of surgical educational applications using AR and VR technology that aim to improve anatomic conceptualization and simulate surgical procedures to improve clinical performance. Understanding of anatomic structures is essential in the surgical training of all specialties and for performing some complex unusual operations. Randomized controlled trials have demonstrated significantly superior identification of key anatomic features with faster responses by trainees who were provided with 3-dimensional (3D) images compared with 2D images in different specialties, especially amongst women.[3,4] AR superimposes additional data over real images in 3D, enhancing the spatial presentation and enabling exploration of various anatomic models

Disclosure Statement: Dr C. Cao has nothing to disclose. Dr R.J. Cerfolio discloses relationships with Bovie, Community Health Services, Covidien/Medtronic, C-SATS, Davol/Bard, Ethicon, Google/Verb, Intuitive Surgical, KCI/Acelity Company, Myriad Genetics, Pinnacle, ROLO-7 Consulting Firm, and TEGO Corporation.
[a] Department of Cardiothoracic Surgery, New York University Langone Health, 530 1st Avenue, 9V, New York, NY 10016, USA; [b] Department of Cardiothoracic Surgery, New York University Langone Health, 550 1st Avenue, 15th Floor, New York, NY 10016, USA
* Corresponding author.
E-mail address: Robert.Cerfolio@nyulangone.org
; @Cerf_MD (R.J.C.)

thoracic.theclinics.com

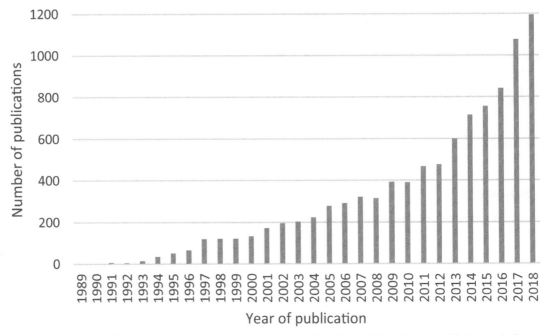

Fig. 1. Number of publications on virtual reality or augmented reality published in scientific journals. (www. pubmed.com.)

using real-life images through portable mobile devices or head-mounted display systems.[5,6] An example of anatomic education through 3D imaging is the Anatomage Virtual Dissection Table (Anatomage, San Jose, California, USA), which displays holographic projections of organs onto a touch screen table.[6] Benefits of these 3D programs and their interactive platforms have translated into improved learning and positive feedback from students.[3,7]

In addition to the 3D display of anatomic structures, both AR and VR technology have been used to recreate digital or superimposed environments to resemble immersive surgical procedures or scenarios for educational purposes. VR programs are able to generate 3D images with interactive features such as tactile feedback, which enables the trainee to simulate procedures that are designed to reduce the learning curve and facilitate tactile learning.[8] A recent systematic review on AR technology used in medical training identified 26 studies involving various simulators, which were categorized into laparoscopic tasks, neurosurgical procedures, and echocardiography training.[9] Specific examples of laparoscopic simulators included instrumentation systems that assessed the motion control, navigation, positioning, suturing, dissection, and knot tying skills of the trainee.[10] Neurosurgical procedures included ultrasound-guided joint injections using a platform that overlaid AR imaging over phantom models.[11,12] Randomized controlled trials

comparing these platforms with a controlled group reported significantly higher success rate and lower injury rate in the AR group by participating residents.[11,12] Despite these encouraging findings, Barsom and colleagues[9] noted a lack of follow-up of these studies to assess the retention of skills acquired from AR applications and a lack of evidence to demonstrate a translation to improvement in patient clinical outcomes. Nonetheless, the investigators postulated that AR will help to bridge the gap between attaining procedural skills in the real clinical setting by training them in a virtual context. An excellent example of this was demonstrated by Calatayud and colleagues,[13] who reported superior surgical performance by surgeons who completed a brief VR "warm up" program before laparoscopic cholecystectomy, compared with surgeons who did not.

There is now growing evidence from randomized controlled trials that AR and VR simulators provide significant improvements in the accuracy, safety, and speed of performing certain surgical tasks by residents.[14,15] These simulators also offer reliable and objective measurement of performance metrics that can be repeated between trainees and over time, providing valuable data that can be analyzed to optimize curricula and assess individual performance. Furthermore, the use of simulators avoids some of the challenges associated with traditional cadaveric teaching models, such as their limited numbers and potential infection risks. To further validate AR and VR applications as truly effective educational tools, several assessments need to be examined in future studies. These included *face validity*, the degree to which an AR application resembles the real working situation; *content validity*, which refers to the educational content of the application; *construct validity*, which is the degree to which results of a training session as performed by the trainee using the AR application reflect the actual skill of the trainee; *concurrent validity*, which measures the improvement in performance using the application in comparison to a preexisting training method; and *predictive validity*, the degree of concordance between outcomes in the AR application and in reality.[9,16] Further development of AR and VR simulators should aim to systematically report these end points to scientifically assess the efficacy of these applications as educational tools. Examples of existing clinical and educational uses of AR and VR technology in different surgical specialties are presented in **Tables 1** and **2**, respectively.

Beyond education and training, the use of AR and VR technology is already a reality in patient care through several clinical applications, particularly in preoperative surgical planning and intraoperative navigation. Over the past half century, the expansion and evolution of imaging techniques have far outpaced their display platforms. Imaging modalities such as PET, computed tomography (CT), and MRI have become widespread preoperative investigations, enabling the physician to analyze complex conditions in ever increasing detail with greater accuracy and less invasiveness. Despite these advanced techniques and the additional data they contribute to the diagnosis and planning of procedures, the display of these images have largely been limited to 2D imaging on conventional computer screens. It has been estimated that 118 million image-guided surgeries are performed worldwide each year, with 21 million within the United States alone.[6] With the development of AR and VR technology, clinical information such as medical imaging, patient data, and procedural details can be projected more effectively and efficiently to benefit surgical planning, reduce operative time, and improve the operative experience for the surgeon.[17] AR is able to achieve this by overlaying additional computer-generated data over the real-life operative field, providing an enriched "fusion" view for the surgeon in real time through devices such as the headset.

To examine the clinical evidence in this field, Yoon and colleagues[6] performed a systematic review on the head-up display platforms in current use, including the Google Glass (Google, Mountain View, California, USA) and the Sony stereoscopic

head-mounted display systems (Sony, Tokyo, Japan). These devices allow live streaming from endoscopy, navigation images from intraoperative MRI or CT, and display of preoperative imaging. Other platforms such as HoloLens (Microsoft, Redmond, Washington, USA) enables the user to see holograms of preprogrammed images in their line of vision, with potential for seeing 3D reconstructions from preoperative images overlaid onto the real surgical field.[6] Metrics used to assess the usefulness of these devices typically included subjective pre- and postoperative surveys from the surgeon, as well as objective measurements such as time spend for a particular procedure with or without the head device. Specific examples of clinical use for AR display systems include live streaming of fluoroscopy during spinal surgery,[18] display of neuroendoscopy videos during neurosurgery,[19] concurrent viewing of cardiopulmonary data during cardiothoracic surgery,[20] and 4D visualization of optical coherence tomography in ophthalmology surgery.[21] Challenges identified in the field of AR and VR display units include physical hardware limitations, such as the size and comfort of the devices and limitation of battery life, software limitations such as suboptimal voice recognition and data streaming, potential distraction of certain displays, and privacy concerns related to encryption and coding.[6]

A research area of intense focus has been the use of AR and VR technology for intraoperative navigation. Concurrent use of AR and VR display systems with traditional imaging techniques have shown encouraging results to suggest reduced risks and improved safety for surgical procedures.[22–24] Examples of this include the use of an AR platform consisting of a magnetic tracking system with integrated sensors to project virtual representations of the heart onto transesophageal echocardiogram during mitral valve repair surgery.[22] Using this novel AR technology on porcine models, the investigators were able to demonstrate fewer errors, shorter navigation times, and higher success rates when using the AR platform compared with using transesophageal echocardiogram alone.[22] The use of AR technology in preoperative planning and intraoperative navigation has also been demonstrated in neurosurgery. Low and colleagues[23] used a stereoscopic 3D planning system that enabled the identification of intricate intracranial structures surrounding the tumor using preoperative MRI data, allowing the surgeon to manipulate the tissues in a 3D VR workstation the day before surgery to plan their incisional approach. The use of AR technology was further used intraoperatively, overlaying the preoperative images onto the surgical field in

Table 1
Examples of augmented reality and virtual reality technology currently in use for clinical applications in different surgical specialties

Specialty Education	VR or AR Technique	Uses	Benefits	Challenges	Future Direction
Dentistry	AR simulator for training and OSCE examination[26]	Tracking system enables handpiece and screen synchronization	Evaluation of ergonomic postures, improves hand-eye coordination Decrease faculty interaction time by 5-fold[27] Ability to program different scenarios Objective assessment tools for procedural tasks[28]	Development of standardized learning curricula	Educational curricula and standardized assessments
Laparoscopic surgery	Anatomic surgical anatomy of liver surgery[3,29] ProMIS AR simulator for laparoscopic procedures[10] Training for laparoscopic liver resection[30]	Training and assessment of laparoscopic tasks, eg, navigation, positioning, suturing, dissection, knot tying	Haptic feedback Useful assessment tool High face validity and construct validity[9]	Reduction in cost of commercially available systems	Increased availability for surgical trainees by decreasing costs
Cardiology	AR headset connected to ultrasound probe to simulate echocardiographic views on mannequin[1]	The operator visualizes the AR anatomic perspective that is superimposed on the virtual simulator	No risk to patients Multiple trainees with one trainer Connectivity at different locations through network Generated true 3D image to enhance anatomic correlation	Cost associated with hardware; limited vision of VR headset and physical size; limited connectivity in long distances	Improved hardware and software associated with headset platform

Specialty	Simulator type	Applications	Benefits	Challenges	Future directions
Spine surgery	AR- and VR-based simulators[2,11]	Simulation for pedicle screw placement, vertebroplasty, posterior cervical laminectomy and foraminotomy, lumbar puncture, facet joint injection, and spinal needle insertion and placement	Improved trainee skills, accuracy, speed Reliable, objective measurement of performance metrics	Accuracy of haptic feedback mechanisms	Development of standardized simulation curricula[2]
Neurosurgery	Task-oriented simulators with haptic feedback	Ventricular catheter insertion Ventriculoperitoneal shunt insertion[31] Base of skull bone drilling exercises[32]	Avoidance of expense, availability, and infection risks associated with cadavers	Improvement in registration, tracking, and calibration in simulators	Further maturation in simulator development
Ophthalmic surgery	VR simulator	Cataract surgery exercises involving an objective-structured assessment tool to assess technical skills at various steps of the procedure[33]	Significantly improved performance scores in novice and intermediate-level surgeons according to randomized controlled trials[33]	Correlation of performance assessments to clinical outcomes in patients	Objective data to support improvement in clinical outcomes

Abbreviation: OSCE, objective structured clinical examination.

Table 2
Examples of augmented reality and virtual reality technology currently in use for surgical education in different surgical specialties

Specialty Clinical Care	VR or AR Technique	Uses	Benefits	Challenges	Future Direction
Hepatobiliary surgery	Overlay of virtual 3D images onto real-time surgical field AR-assisted intraoperative navigation[34]	Real-time visualization of intrahepatic structures, blood vessels, and tumors Virtual images of organs and lesions compensate for surgeon's lack of tactile sensation in videoscopic procedures[34] Identification of tumor location and margins in robotic surgery[35,36] Roles in open surgery, percutaneous surgery, and autotransplantation[34]	Improves accuracy of resections and identification of intrahepatic structures Real-time overlay overcomes variations such as ventilation movements	Liver transformation and registration errors during surgery	Improved fusion of multiple imaging modalities Improved biomechanical liver modeling Enhanced image data processing
Neurosurgery	Fusion of MRI, MRA and CT brain images to digital microscopy[8,37] Computer-assisted navigation to provide intraoperative image guidance Head-mount display to aid in neuroendoscopy[19]	Overlay of AR images to provide additional data to surgical field Display of acquired 3D images in magnification and over multiple monitors[8] Surgical planning using integrated images and projecting as 3D volumetric objects Improved visualization in pituitary adenoma and other intracranial resections	AR able to guide instruments, visualize target, avoid crucial anatomic structures such as vessels Reduced visual strain	Current navigation systems still require some shifting of focus between surgical field and navigation display	AR combined with artificial intelligence to provide real-time surgical navigation to provide real-time overlay of 3D anatomy over a surgical field, visualizing critical structures and tracking instruments[8]

Specialty	Technology	Application	Benefits	Limitations	Future directions
Ophthalmic surgery	VR simulator for cataract surgery Head-up display of optical coherence tomography and vitreoretinal imaging with 3D glasses[6,38]	Phacoemulsifications and vitrectomies Visualization of cataract or retina	Avoidance of switching views by the surgeon Improved accuracy of simulated corneal suture placement[21] Higher success rate and shorter operative time[38]	Limited image illumination	Improvement in the brightness of newer models
Orthopedic surgery	Overlay of fluoroscopy or electromyogram signals during spinal surgery through head-mounted systems[6,18]	Spinal surgery Pedicle screw placement	Shorter operative time[13] Reduced radiation exposure for the surgeon	Live streaming of video data due to wireless network technology	Development of more secure data processing networks
Urology	Display of live endoscopic video through head-mounted system in real time	Radical nephrectomy, nephroureterectomy, urethral stents, prostate cancer[39,40]	Improved visualization of ureteric structures during stenting and resection	Ergonomics of headgear in long operations[40] Shifting of focus	Improving physical comfort of head-up devices Development of holographic projections to avoid shifting of focus
Interventional cardiology	3D overlay of TEE, CMRI, and CT images onto live fluoroscopy 3D digital heart model displayed with a separate, stand-alone viewer	Identification of specific anatomic targets when closing intracardiac defects Selection of gantry angles for optimal procedural guidance and provision of continuous roadmap Design of individualized and customized devices[41]	Decrease procedure times Decrease radiation exposure[42]	Significant learning curve and expertise in cardiac pathology and imaging	Improved display platforms to enable more complex percutaneous repair interventions

Abbreviations: CMRI, cardiovascular MRI; CT, computed tomography; MRA, magnetic resonance angiography; TEE, transesophageal echocardiogram.

real-time, thus improving the conceptualization of the tumor location in 3D, akin to "x-ray" vision for the surgeon. The investigators successfully applied this strategy in 5 patients who underwent surgical excision of meningiomas. Other examples of the use of AR and VR technology in intraoperative navigation can be found in intrahepatic radiofrequency ablation and endobronchial photodynamic therapy procedures.[24,25]

In summary, there are many applications of AR and VR technology in surgical education and surgical planning, concentrated on 3D conceptualization, procedural simulation, and intraoperative navigation. The improved projection of anatomic structures in 3D have been shown to be more effective than traditional flat screen imaging for students, whereas immersive simulations have improved the performance of procedures by surgical trainees and surgeons in a variety of specialties.[3,14] The use of AR technology by superimposing preoperative and intraoperative images onto a live surgical field have enabled the surgeon to visualize critical structures that are not visible by direct vision.[22,23] To validate the effectiveness of these applications, researchers have developed objective assessments to analyze the effectiveness of educational tools and navigation systems.[9] Future studies will aim to directly correlate the utilization of these applications to the clinical outcomes of patients. It can be foreseen that the translation of improved AR and VR technologies into improved clinical outcomes will further accelerate the development in this exciting field.

REFERENCES

1. Mahmood F, Mahmood E, Dorfman RG, et al. Augmented reality and ultrasound education: initial experience. J Cardiothorac Vasc Anesth 2018;32: 1363–7.

2. Pfandler M, Lazarovici M, Stefan P, et al. Virtual reality-based simulators for spine surgery: a systematic review. Spine J 2017;17:1352–63.

3. Muller-Stich BP, Lob N, Wald D, et al. Regular three-dimensional presentations improve in the identification of surgical liver anatomy - a randomized study. BMC Med Educ 2013;13:131.

4. Prinz A, Bolz M, Findl O. Advantage of three dimensional animated teaching over traditional surgical videos for teaching ophthalmic surgery: a randomised study. Br J Ophthalmol 2005;89:1495–9.

5. Jain N, Youngblood P, Hasel M, et al. An augmented reality tool for learning spatial anatomy on mobile devices. Clin Anat 2017;30:736–41.

6. Yoon JW, Chen RE, Kim EJ, et al. Augmented reality for the surgeon: systematic review. Int J Med Robot 2018;14:e1914.

7. Kurniawan MS, Witjaksono S, Witjaksono D, et al. Human anatomy learning systems using augmented reality on mobile application. Procedia Comput Sci 2018;135:80–8.

8. Bernardo A. Virtual reality and simulation in neurosurgical training. World Neurosurg 2017;106: 1015–29.

9. Barsom EZ, Graafland M, Schijven MP. Systematic review on the effectiveness of augmented reality applications in medical training. Surg Endosc 2016;30: 4174–83.

10. Botden SM, Jakimowicz JJ. What is going on in augmented reality simulation in laparoscopic surgery? Surg Endosc 2009;23:1693–700.

11. Moult E, Ungi T, Welch M, et al. Ultrasound-guided facet joint injection training using Perk Tutor. Int J Comput Assist Radiol Surg 2013;8:831–6.

12. Keri Z, Sydor D, Ungi T, et al. Computerized training system for ultrasound-guided lumbar puncture on abnormal spine models: a randomized controlled trial. Can J Anaesth 2015;62:777–84.

13. Calatayud D, Arora S, Aggarwal R, et al. Warm-up in a virtual reality environment improves performance in the operating room. Ann Surg 2010;251:1181–5.

14. Chaer RA, Derubertis BG, Lin SC, et al. Simulation improves resident performance in catheter-based intervention: results of a randomized, controlled study. Ann Surg 2006;244:343–52.

15. Seymour NE, Gallagher AG, Roman SA, et al. Virtual reality training improves operating room performance: results of a randomized, double-blinded study. Ann Surg 2002;236:458–63 [discussion: 463–4].

16. van Dongen KW, Tournoij E, van der Zee DC, et al. Construct validity of the LapSim: can the LapSim virtual reality simulator distinguish between novices and experts? Surg Endosc 2007;21:1413–7.

17. Yoon JW, Chen RE, ReFaey K, et al. Technical feasibility and safety of image-guided parieto-occipital ventricular catheter placement with the assistance of a wearable head-up display. Int J Med Robot 2017;13. https://doi.org/10.1002/rcs.1836.

18. Yoon JW, Chen RE, Han PK, et al. Technical feasibility and safety of an intraoperative head-up display device during spine instrumentation. Int J Med Robot 2017;13. https://doi.org/10.1002/rcs.1770.

19. Levy ML, Day JD, Albuquerque F, et al. Heads-up intraoperative endoscopic imaging: a prospective evaluation of techniques and limitations. Neurosurgery 1997;40:526–30 [discussion: 530–1].

20. Austin JW. Evaluation of a "heads-up" display for cardiopulmonary bypass. J Extra Corpor Technol 2000; 32:49–53.

21. Carrasco-Zevallos OM, Keller B, Viehland C, et al. Live volumetric (4D) visualization and guidance of in vivo human ophthalmic surgery with intraoperative optical coherence tomography. Sci Rep 2016;6: 31689.

22. Chu MW, Moore J, Peters T, et al. Augmented reality image guidance improves navigation for beating heart mitral valve repair. Innovations (Phila) 2012;7: 274–81.

23. Low D, Lee CK, Dip LL, et al. Augmented reality neurosurgical planning and navigation for surgical excision of parasagittal, falcine and convexity meningiomas. Br J Neurosurg 2010;24: 69–74.

24. Fuchs H, State A, Yang H, et al. Optimizing a head-tracked stereo display system to guide hepatic tumor ablation. Stud Health Technol Inform 2008;132: 126–31.

25. Yoon SH, Goo JM, Lee CH, et al. Virtual reality-assisted localization and three-dimensional printing-enhanced multidisciplinary decision to treat radiologically occult superficial endobronchial lung cancer. Thorac Cancer 2018;9(11):1525–7.

26. Roy E, Bakr MM, George R. The need for virtual reality simulators in dental education: a review. Saudi Dent J 2017;29:41–7.

27. Jasinevicius TR, Landers M, Nelson S, et al. An evaluation of two dental simulation systems: virtual reality versus contemporary non-computer-assisted. J Dent Educ 2004;68:1151–62.

28. Huang TK, Yang CH, Hsieh YH, et al. Augmented reality (AR) and virtual reality (VR) applied in dentistry. Kaohsiung J Med Sci 2018;34:243–8.

29. Beermann J, Tetzlaff R, Bruckner T, et al. Three-dimensional visualisation improves understanding of surgical liver anatomy. Med Educ 2010;44: 936–40.

30. Strickland A, Fairhurst K, Lauder C, et al. Development of an ex vivo simulated training model for laparoscopic liver resection. Surg Endosc 2011;25: 1677–82.

31. Robison RA, Liu CY, Apuzzo ML. Man, mind, and machine: the past and future of virtual reality simulation in neurologic surgery. World Neurosurg 2011; 76:419–30.

32. Wiet GJ, Schmalbrock P, Powell K, et al. Use of ultrahigh-resolution data for temporal bone dissection simulation. Otolaryngol Head neck Surg 2005;133: 911–5.

33. Thomsen AS, Bach-Holm D, Kjaerbo H, et al. Operating room performance improves after proficiency-based virtual reality cataract surgery training. Ophthalmology 2017;124:524–31.

34. Tang R, Ma LF, Rong ZX, et al. Augmented reality technology for preoperative planning and intraoperative navigation during hepatobiliary surgery: a review of current methods. Hepatobiliary Pancreat Dis Int 2018;17:101–12.

35. Buchs NC, Volonte F, Pugin F, et al. Augmented environments for the targeting of hepatic lesions during image-guided robotic liver surgery. J Surg Res 2013;184:825–31.

36. Pessaux P, Diana M, Soler L, et al. Towards cybernetic surgery: robotic and augmented reality-assisted liver segmentectomy. Langenbecks Arch Surg 2015;400:381–5.

37. Levitt MR, Ghodke BV, Cooke DL, et al. Endovascular procedures with CTA and MRA roadmapping. J Neuroimaging 2011;21:259–62.

38. Shen L, Carrasco-Zevallos O, Keller B, et al. Novel microscope-integrated stereoscopic heads-up display for intrasurgical optical coherence tomography. Biomed Opt Express 2016;7:1711–26.

39. Yoshida S, Kihara K, Takeshita H, et al. Head-mounted display for a personal integrated image monitoring system: ureteral stent placement. Urol Int 2015;94:117–20.

40. Yoshida S, Kihara K, Takeshita H, et al. A head-mounted display-based personal integrated-image monitoring system for transurethral resection of the prostate. Wideochir Inne Tech Maloinwazyjne 2014; 9:644–9.

41. Olivieri L, Krieger A, Chen MY, et al. 3D heart model guides complex stent angioplasty of pulmonary venous baffle obstruction in a Mustard repair of D-TGA. Int J Cardiol 2014;172:e297–8.

42. Grant EK, Olivieri LJ. The role of 3-D heart models in planning and executing interventional procedures. Can J Cardiol 2017;33:1074–81.

Artificial Intelligence
Can Information be Transformed into Intelligence in Surgical Education?

Ahmad Y. Sheikh, MD[a,b,*], James I. Fann, MD[c]

KEYWORDS

- Surgery • Education • Artificial intelligence • Machine learning • Patient safety

KEY POINTS

- Early application of artificial intelligence (AI) technologies has been in those specialties that are predominantly image based or visually based.
- Procedure-based specialties, such as surgery, may require a longer time before realizing operational AI technology.
- A potential application of AI in surgical education is as a teaching coach or mentor that interacts with the user via virtual and/or augmented reality.
- To drive the development of AI in education will require demonstrated improvement in patient safety and outcomes.
- The question arises as to whether machines will achieve the wisdom and intelligence of a human educator.

INTRODUCTION

In 1968, the award-winning director Stanley Kubrick introduced to the audience a vision of a dystopian future in *2001: A Space Odyssey*. In the film, the artificial intelligence (AI) entity HAL 9000 (Heuristically programmed ALgorithmic computer) was advanced enough to be sentient and to plot against its creators to ensure self-preservation.[1] Although the year 2001 has come and gone and no HAL—as originally conceived—has yet emerged, we are living in a time where we speak to smart-home hubs, allow cars to drive themselves, and rely on the predictive analytics of smartphones to navigate daily concerns, such as traffic routes. Many experts posit that a technological singularity is likely in the next 50 years, whereby conglomeration of technology will enter a reaction of self-improvement cycles and thus exceed human intelligence. Whether or not we will live to see this singularity remains in speculation; however, it is clear that AI is beginning to have an impact on all aspects of the human condition, including how medicine is practiced and taught.

In 2016 alone, the McKinsey Global Institute estimated a global investment of $26 billion to $39 billion in AI-based technology, with the bulk of the funds provided by tech giants, such as Google.[2] Up to $9 billion of the total was attributed to start-up and more nimble companies. The health care industry makes up a minority of this ecosystem, much of which has been directed at diagnostics and therapy. Although AI technologies have advanced rapidly in many fields, their

Disclosure Statement: The authors have nothing to disclose.
[a] Division of Cardiothoracic Surgery, Kaiser Permanente, 2238 Geary Boulevard, 8th Floor, San Francisco, CA 94115, USA; [b] Division of Cardiothoracic Surgery, University of California, San Francisco, CA, USA; [c] Department of Cardiothoracic Surgery, Stanford University, 300 Pasteur Drive, CVRB, Stanford, CA 94305, USA
* Corresponding author. Division of Cardiothoracic Surgery, Kaiser Permanente, 2238 Geary Blvd, 8th floor, San Francisco, CA 94115.
E-mail address: ahmad.y.sheikh@kp.org

Thorac Surg Clin 29 (2019) 339–350
https://doi.org/10.1016/j.thorsurg.2019.03.011

implementation in patient care settings has yet to become widespread.[3–10] Nonetheless, AI offers opportunity for substantial transformation, particularly with respect to more effective training of health care providers.

This article reviews the fundamentals of AI, provides a background of AI in the medical field, and postulates how AI can specifically have an impact on surgical practices and education in the future. It also describes a brief vignette, a glimpse into the future to illustrate how AI technologies may be implemented within the next decade or so.

ARTIFICIAL INTELLIGENCE AND INTELLIGENCE AGENTS

In its broadest and simplest sense, AI may be defined as intelligence manifested by machines and the development of algorithms, as opposed to the natural intelligence possessed by biologically evolved organisms.[3,5,6,11–13] It is the capacity of a machine to perform functions analogous to human learning and decision making. To achieve this level of intelligence, machines (or computers) utilize intelligence agents, which are sensors and devices that perceive environments and take actions that maximize chances of successfully achieving goals.[3,4,10,12,14–16] The earliest demonstration of AI appears to be in 1956 at a computing conference held at Dartmouth College.[16] There, rudimentary algorithms were developed that enabled computers to play checkers, solve basic algebra equations, and "speak" in English. It was one of the inventors of the early checker programs, Arthur Samuel, who in 1959 coined the term, *machine learning*.[17]

The modern spectrum of intelligence agents ranges from the simplest of devices, such as thermostats, to complex multilayered neural networks designed to recapitulate an organism's general (and eventually specific) thought processes.[3,4,13,15] As can be imagined, the field of AI draws un multiple disciplines, technologies, and philosophies as well as learning and behavioral theories (**Fig. 1**). In medicine, early application of AI technologies are likely those specialties that are predominantly image based or visually based, such as radiology, pathology, ophthalmology, and dermatology.[5,6,8,10,13,18–24] Procedure-based specialties, such as surgery, may require a longer time before fully realizing operational AI technologies, partly due to the complex nature of interactions with human tissues and the perceived lack of evidence and awareness of the potential of computational approaches.[5,6,8,25] Regarding surgical practice, the current vision of AI is to augment and complement the surgeon, particularly regarding surgical decision making and particular components of operative surgery.

DOMAINS OF ARTIFICIAL INTELLIGENCE

Reviews of AI in surgery highlight basic subfields well recognized in AI research: machine learning (including artificial neural networks), natural language processing, and computer perception and vision.[3–5,8–10,12,13,25] These fields overlap with additional domains, such as social and general intelligence.

At the outset, the idea is that AI is a term representative of leading-edge technology. That is, today's routine predictive computational algorithms (eg, smartphone-suggested travel routes to minimize transit time) were yesterday's AI. This is known as the AI effect, whereby once a problem is solved by AI, the solution is no longer considered intelligent.[26] The classic example is the IBM chess computer Deep Blue. Once Deep Blue defeated the chess champion Garry Kasparov in 1996, there was much debate as to whether the machine actually demonstrated intelligence versus brute-force computing. Thus, despite innumerable intelligence agents already deployed in everyday workflows, they may not be referred to as AI.[26] Similarly, once the technologies covered in this article become routine in the future, they likely will not be thought of as part of the AI domain.

Machine learning is perhaps the most fundamental subset of all AI domains, providing a basic foundation for intelligence agents to function (**Fig. 2**).[3–6,8–10,12,13,18,25] In its purest sense, machine learning is the discipline that focuses on how computers learn from data and develop predictions in novel situations from previous observations.[5,12,25] Pattern recognition is the heart of machine learning; thus, the algorithm within machine learning relies on data collection and input to achieve the task.[5,7,9] There are 3 major categories of machine learning: supervised, unsupervised, and reinforcement learning. In all cases, the machine makes predictions, or interprets, the data in the absence of explicit programming, hence the "intelligence" of the system (**Fig. 3**).[3–6,8–10,12,18,25]

In supervised machine learning, the objective is defined beforehand and the machine begins with a goal of predicting a known output.[3,5,12,25] Often, the algorithm attempts to mimic the ability of a highly trained individual with domain expertise, for example, a physician skilled in diagnostic testing. One example of current supervised machine learning in medicine is the automated ECG interpretation, which exists in many commercially

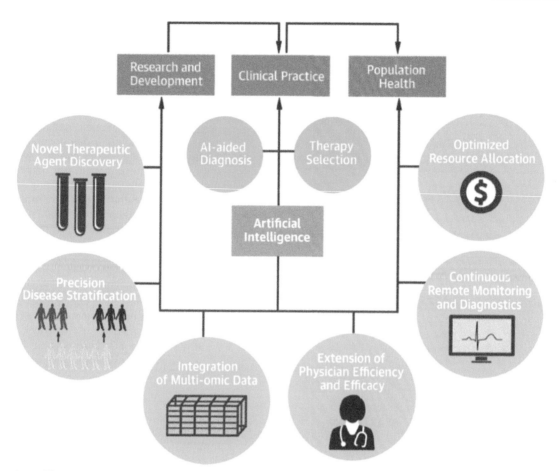

Fig. 1. The Incorporation of AI into cardiovascular medicine will affect all aspects of cardiology, from research and development to clinical practice to population health. The figure shows selected applications within all 3 domains of cardiovascular care. (*From* Johnson KW, Torres Soto J, Glicksberg BS, et al. Artificial intelligence in cardiology. J Am Coll Cardiol 2018;71:2670.)

available ECG machines.[3,12] In this case, there is a set number of diagnoses or interpretations, such as myocardial ischemia and ventricular arrhythmias, and the machine interprets the data to determine if the diagnosis exists and is applicable.

Unsupervised learning, in contrast, does not specify or define an output or target.[3–6,8,9,12,25] In this type of learning, the computer looks for patterns or groupings within the data. This approach may be especially useful for detecting subtle patterns in large data sets, such as in facilitating analysis of big data. An example of such algorithms utilized in medical research includes ontological genomic data analysis, that is, defining how the data points are represented and their relationships. In a clinical study demonstrating unsupervised learning, application of a machine learning algorithm correctly identified surgical site infections with a high degree of sensitivity and specificity.[27] Similarly, other investigators used a machine learning model to predict with accuracy

deep incisional site infections using blood test data after gastrointestinal surgery.[28]

The third domain of machine learning is reinforcement learning, in which the input and outputs pairs are not specified, and the focus of the machine is to perform a task while learning from its own successes and mistakes to improve its performance (**Fig. 4**).[3,5,10,13,29] This type of algorithm is akin to biological homeostasis, where numerous series of biofeedback loops help regulate a physiologic parameter, such as blood sodium levels. Reinforcement learning algorithms have been proposed for the development of artificial organ systems, such as an artificial pancreas, which in a closed-loop fashion can fine-tune its measurement of blood glucose and delivery of insulin[5,29]

As the applications for machine learning have become multidimensional, so too have the computing methods evolved in complexity. One example of advanced computing inspired by biological systems is the idea of artificial neural

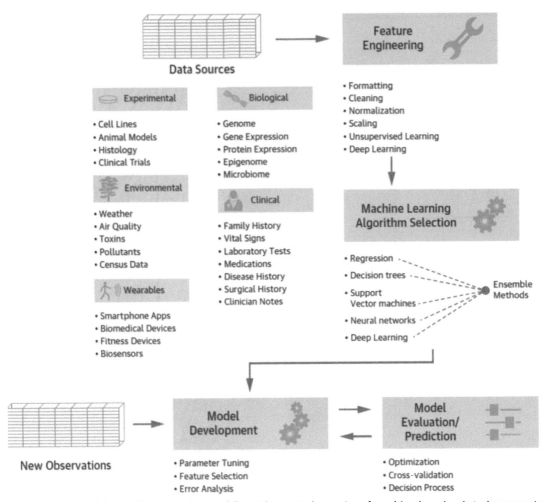

Fig. 2. Overview of the machine learning workflow. The central promise of machine learning is to incorporate data from a variety of sources (clinical measurements and observations, biological omics, experimental results, environmental information, and wearable devices) into sensible models for describing and predicting human disease. The typical machine learning workflow begins with data acquisition, proceeds to feature engineering and then to algorithm selection and model development, and finally results in model evaluation and application. (*From* Johnson KW, Torres Soto J, Glicksberg BS, et al. Artificial intelligence in cardiology. J Am Coll Cardiol 2018;71:2671.)

networks involved in deep learning. In these systems, "neurons" are composed of simple computational units (**Fig. 5**).[3–5,9,10,12,13,25] These neurons synapse with one another at nodes, where inputs and outputs are weighted to adjust the learning process. Complexity of the network increases as additional "layers" of neurons are added, such that deep learning networks can be created. Such neural networks can be applied to image recognition, risk prediction, voice recognition, and medical diagnostics. Much like their biological counterparts, although neural networks can perform at a high accuracy, the exact algorithms by which the such a network achieves its tasks remain deeply embedded in the layers of the network. Thus, although the network can accomplish a task, it may be difficult and perhaps impossible to retrace how the network processed the information. Regardless, deep learning networks are showing promise in medical applications, such as outcome prediction for patients undergoing heart transplantation.[30]

With machine learning as the predominant AI domain, other subfields also have translational relevance to surgical education. Computer perception (including image recognition) is the element of computers recognizing those environmental stimuli, which the human brain has evolved to interpret as part of daily existence.[2,5,13] Perceptive domains can include images, sounds, scenes,

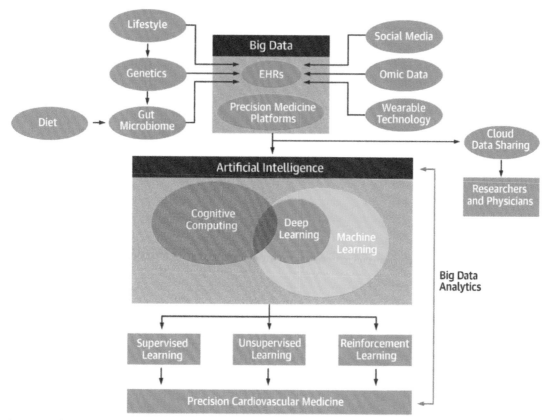

Fig. 3. Big data (genetics, social media, environmental, and lifestyle-related factors, or omics data) can be stored through electronic health records (EHRs) or precision medicine platforms and can be shared for data analysis and other physicians or researchers through secure cloud systems. Big data analytics using AI (machine learning, deep learning, or cognitive computing) and 3 main types of learning algorithms (supervised, unsupervised, and reinforcement learning) will enable precision cardiovascular medicine. (*From* Kittanawong C, Zhang HJ, Wang Z, et al. Artificial intelligence in precision cardiovascular medicine. J Am Coll Cardiol 2017;69:2662; with permission.)

and language. Natural language processing is a domain onto itself, whereby machines can learn to understand human language in processing and analyzing a large amount of data.[2,5,10,13,31] Examples of this technology include scraping electronic health records to extract and interpret data from practitioners' written content. As might be imagined, this requires more than simple word recognition but complex and nuanced appreciation of the lexicon, syntax, and context. Examples of natural language processing in the current state include the ability to predict anastomotic leaks by processing operative reports and progress notes in an electronic health record.[31]

Similar to natural language processing, image recognition requires computers to learn how to perceive, categorize, and analyze images that the human brain processes naturally.[2,5,9,10] More than simple pattern recognition, deep learning networks can be called on to sift through visual data and make meaningful interpretations much like

a human domain expert. As AI engines have developed, it has become clear that integration and overlap of various domains are required to achieve pragmatic efficacy. To achieve meaningful output, AI constructs often might require a combination of artificial neural networks, machine learning, and perceptive abilities.[2,5,9,10] With the digitization of medical data, large sets of pathologic and radiographic images are now available; thus, computer-assisted diagnosis with machine learning has been at the forefront of technological innovation.[5,9,10,18,19] Machine learning has been used to detect lymph node metastasis in breast cancer in slide images, in some cases achieving better diagnostic performance than expert pathologists.[19] In radiology, there have been advances in automated machine learning systems to detect and characterize lung nodules.[10,22] Using a deep learning algorithm applied to image analysis based on a data set of 128,175 retinal fundus photographs, Gulshan and colleagues[21] reported high

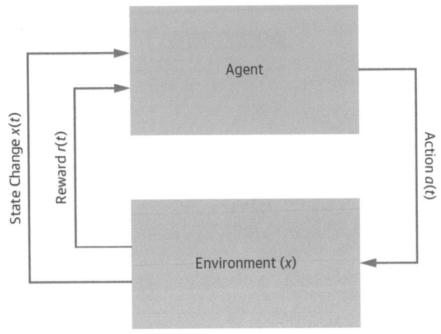

Fig. 4. Reinforcement learning algorithms are used to train the action of an agent on an environment. (*From* Johnson KW, Torres Soto J, Glicksberg BS, et al. Artificial intelligence in cardiology. J Am Coll Cardiol 2018;71:2674.)

sensitivity and specificity for detecting diabetic retinopathy for ophthalmologic referral. The Food and Drug Administration recently approved the marketing of an AI-based diagnostic device IDx-DR (IDx, Coralville, IA), which detects diabetic retinopathy.[32] Taken with a retinal camera, images of the eye are analyzed to determine whether diabetic retinopathy is present; IDx-DR is the first device approved for marketing that provides a screening decision without the need for a clinician to interpret the results.[32] A direct application of image processing and deep learning in surgical education comes from Stanford University School of Medicine, where the intent is to be able to assess surgical or technical proficiency.[33]

Despite promising results, it is unlikely that AI systems will replace physicians any time soon; instead, they will enhance human performance and lessen the burden of repetitive tasks.[9,10] In doing so, it is critical to continue to review and interrogate AI algorithms. Based on a data set of 129,450 images of cutaneous lesions with known diagnoses, Esteva and colleagues[23] trained a neural network to differentiate between benign and malignant skin lesions based on appearance and found that its performance was comparable to that of expert dermatologists in diagnosing a limited set of cutaneous lesions. Because AI algorithms are not explicitly programmed with rules to differentiate benign from malignant cutaneous

lesions, however, they may use unanticipated ways for differentiation. In this study, if an image had a ruler in it, the algorithm was more likely to call it malignant; call it malignant. This was due to the bias in the training data set, because images of lesions that included rulers were more likely to be malignant.[24] Based on 108,948 chest radiographs with disease labels extracted from radiology reports using natural language processing, Wang and colleagues[20] developed an AI algorithm to identify chest pathology, which turned out to be very accurate in identifying pneumothorax. Later analysis suggested, however, that in most chest radiographs that showed a pneumothorax, a chest tube was present.[34] Rather than learning to identify pneumothorax, it is possible that the algorithm learned to identify chest tubes on the radiographs.[34] Thus, for supervised machine learning to work, the training data set must be free of bias; otherwise, such bias may be introduced into the algorithm, diminishing its utility.

INTEGRATING ARTIFICIAL INTELLIGENCE INTO THE REAL WORLD

Traditionally, AI domains help analyze so-called physicalities in the daily world, including medical images, estimation of risk, and even technical or surgical ability. There is an additional aspect to AI, however, which is becoming increasingly

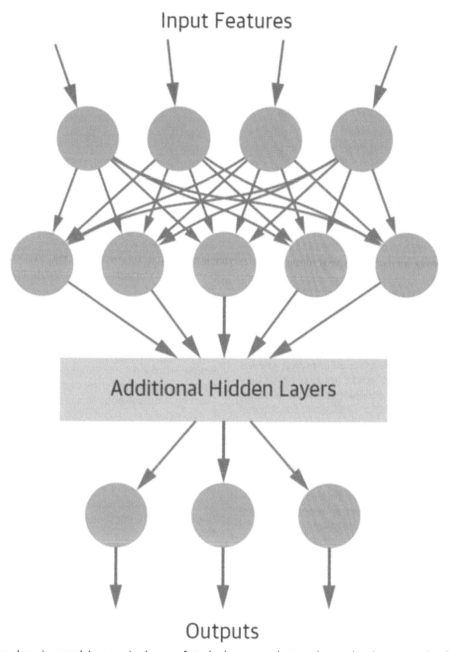

Input Features

Additional Hidden Layers

Outputs

Fig. 5. Deep learning models comprise layers of stacked neurons that can be used to learn complex functions. (*From* Johnson KW, Torres Soto J, Glicksberg BS, et al. Artificial intelligence in cardiology. J Am Coll Cardiol 2018;71:2674.)

crucial if such technology is to be translated into a teaching workflow, namely, social or emotional intelligence with extension into general human intelligence.[2,4,35] Creating intelligence agents that possess the ability to learn social and emotional intelligence is not enough. Such agents will require improved user interfaces to both receive input and interact with humans to generate an output.

Currently, the user interface between machine algorithms and users remains clunky and is not at a level whereby a surgical learner could meaningfully interact with AI engines. There is much progress, however, in introducing more intuitive intelligence engines into everyday workflows; one such element is the idea of chatbots that use AI engines on the backend.

Chatbots are intelligence agents that hover in the background of human lives, listening, analyzing, and ultimately interacting with humans to enable tasks.[2,35] Physicalization of chatbots is evident in smart speakers, such as the Amazon Alexa, or via chat channels on a smartphone. Increasingly, chatbots are utilized to engage humans in a more natural manner than by traditional systems of automated voice prompting. Such health care chatbots can engage patients to improve their care experience; with each interaction, the AI engine gathers more data with regard to what patients need and how workflows might be improved. A potential application for surgical trainees may be similar, whereby a virtual teaching coach is provided in the form of a chatbot.[2,35] Learners may interact with a chatbot that can keep track of their learning, engagement, and progress. On the backend of such a platform, the millions of unique interactions with learners would provide learning footprints, where patterns would be easily detected by the machine learning algorithms. Thus, engagement, assessment, and feedback could be provided to the learner over an extended period. Such a chatbot that resides in a computing cloud could achieve physicality through wearable technology, thus allowing for integration into a realistic educational environment.[35]

Another area where user interface has made great strides is that of virtual or augmented reality visualization.[35–37] Because much of surgical learning relies on visualization and hand-eye coordination, AI engines can interact with a user's visual fields. Augmented reality technology that interactively manipulates displayed information by adding elements of virtual reality is called mixed reality technology.[36] For instance, HoloLens (Microsoft, Redmond, Washington) is a head-mounted mixed reality device that can display a 3-D model or hologram onto the surgical field.[36] Such wearable devices would allow for integrating and presenting information from the various networks to which a learner is connected. This augmented reality technology is a promising initial step; however, visual field interaction will need to become more robust to acquire input (eg, video clips of surgical performance) and provide output (eg, real-time coaching). Current virtual reality headsets are large and obtrusive; future technologies are anticipated to be more streamlined and act as smart glasses. The authors' group's work with the early Google Glass–based telepresence for trainees demonstrated that a wearable technology has potential for improving teaching efficacy in a technical skills environment.[37] Importantly, the ultimate translation of such work would be an AI mentor that could monitor a trainee with smart glasses providing expert level guidance, critique, and review. In terms of improving the educational modalities for the learners, computer vision also can identify signs of the learners' disengagement by monitoring them as they study and work, tracking eye movements and observing their facial expressions to determine whether they are engaged, confused, or bored.[2,5,35]

GLIMPSE INTO THE FUTURE

How might the various concepts integrate into a viable teaching experience for the surgical trainee? The following attempts to capture how AI-enabled teaching tools may transform a learner's experience, not only in documenting progress but also using adaptive learning and personalized teaching. A day in the life of a first-year surgery resident in the not-too-distant future is described.

5:00 AM

The learner awakes and prepares for the day. Her virtual mentor (a combination of a deep neural network, image/video recognition database, and learning progress engine) has culled from the electronic operating room (OR) schedule and the learner's personal calendars what operations and clinical activities are in store for the day. A quick integration across the learner's performance on previous examinations, technical review of her ability in performing operations similar to the upcoming ones, and review of what the learner has read (on electronic format) ensues. The AI engine then physicalizes through a chatbot and speaks to the learner via smart speaker or wearable computing device. This human-like interaction provides the learner with priming educational points for the day and also may include a Socratic teaching moment, whereby important points germane to the day's clinical duties are discussed.

7:00 AM

Rounds (augmented by electronic patient data or health record and decision-making algorithms) are complete, and the AI engine has gathered information from the smart glasses that the learner wears all day, including into the OR. As the first patient is prepared for anesthesia, the learner is receiving information regarding the upcoming operation, reviewing annotated video clips of the learner's past performance in the OR, the simulation laboratory, and other educational environments. Looking through the smart glasses, the learner can review the operation and even perform some of the requisite mechanical motions with the augmentation as the guide.

8:00 *AM*

In the OR, the intelligence agent is continuing to monitor the trainee via the input from the smart glasses and in turn providing teaching points and reminders in the form of pop-up text in the visual field. The interaction between learner, teacher, and other elements in the OR (possibly semiauto-mated robotic assistants) also is captured. Perhaps at one point, the human mentor disables the output of the learning engine as the learner is too distracted. The AI element continues to gather data but does not provide any real-time output to the learner. The learning engine comes back online once the procedure is complete.

12:00 *PM*

During lunch, the AI engine suggests reading and interactive software modules for the learner to complete. The modality switches seamlessly from the wearable device to a tablet or some other communication device. This process facilitates reading the relevant materials and primes the learner for the afternoon clinical duties.

5:00 *PM*

Afternoon rounds commence. The learning engine is integrated into the electronic patient data (or health record) and pertinent vitals, clinical events, and other data are presented in a heads-up fashion via the smart glasses. The learner actively engages the AI engine via voice command to help answer any clinical questions she may have regarding patient management. Each interaction is noted and data gathered are incorporated into the learner's knowledge footprint.

8:00 *PM*

The learner is ready to complete the day. The AI learning engine provides a debriefing displayed on the large monitor at home. Included is a review of any material that the learner inquired about, such as a clinical question, drug dose, or surgical maneuver in the OR. A constructive critique of technical performance in the OR is provided, including video clips captured in the OR. Based on the performance, the AI engine also recommends appropriate future exercises in the simulation laboratory. A review of salient points for next morning's conference also are provided.

PITFALLS AND BARRIERS

Although future projections are compelling, there are many barriers and potential pitfalls in realizing the promise of AI in surgical practice and education.[3–10,12,25] Acknowledging the many technological issues of data storage, integration of electronic data systems, and development of suitable wearable technology, there are issues of accountability regarding patient safety, patient privacy, and transparency related to data management and processing.[3–6,10] Culturally, the idea of a computer being intimately involved in critical decision making in patient care is not appealing to physicians and patients.[5,6] If a patient suffers an adverse event associated with an AI-based technology, there may be multiple sources beyond the health care provider who may be held accountable, including the hardware and software vendors, developers of the algorithms, and sources of the training data.[5,6] Pertaining to diagnosis and treatment recommendations, AI technologies will need transparency in data processing and AI algorithms to determine whether bias has been introduced into the model.[4–6,9] A notable example is the failed application of IBM Watson computer in cancer care.[38] Despite advanced machine learning algorithms and access to large databases, Watson did not fulfill its many expectations. An Achilles heel of AI technologies in health care was apparent in that Watson's treatment recommendations were based on the biases of the physicians who trained it.

An important consideration is the cost of development, implementation, and subsequent payment models of AI-based learning.[5,35] Although there is great incentive for development and application of AI technologies to improve quality and cut costs of patient care, similar incentives may not present for educational applications. To drive the development of AI technologies in education will require demonstrated improvement in patient safety and outcomes. In the short term, implementation of AI teaching tools has the potential to reduce redundancies present in traditional teaching paradigms. For example, if trainees can be prompted in their clinical duties (eg, performing a patient discharge and starting or concluding an operative procedure) by a virtual mentor in real time, efficiency in patient care will likely result. Such efforts, however, would require a dedicated, consolidated effort by the educational community.

Additional issues and challenges will need to be addressed once AI technologies are used in the surgical educational setting. Importantly, the use of AI technologies in training and assessment will require intensive, robust validation, particularly regarding high-stakes summative evaluations. If AI technologies are subject to mistakes and errors, such systems will require continuous monitoring, repairs, and upgrades. The frequency and intensity of auditing and adjudication of AI educational systems will need to be determined. Again, accountability will need to be defined if AI educators and system developers disseminate misinformation or improperly train learners.

ACHIEVING WISDOM AND BEYOND

To date, AI technologies have been used in the medical field by improving clinical workflows, risk assessment, and training. With regard to AI teaching engines, the question arises as to whether machines will achieve the wisdom and intelligence of human educators. As discussed previously, advanced teaching tools may be integrated into surgical education, but none of the current technologies truly replaces multifunctional surgeon educators. Such individuals possess the wisdom of countless years of practice and the technical skills necessary to carry out complex procedures; importantly, they have to be able to impart the knowledge onto learners. Until such requirements are met, it is unlikely that AI technologies will capture the abilities of the surgical educator as an intelligence agent.

One developmental step is that the behaviors of educators could first be captured, and the AI-based assisted behaviors then can be evaluated in the setting of simulation-based training and subsequently in the clinical environment.[11] Currently, the manual interpretations of performance data of educators are possible, but such interpretations are limited by the constraints of retrieval of multimedia data. By employing machine learning algorithms, these observations offer a means to predict and assess high-quality or low-quality performance, in terms of efficiency and error avoidance, and clinical outcome.[11] With advances in robotics, navigation systems, and image-guided interventions, sources of data could be used to train a machine in decision making and assessment.[11,35] The educational paradigm shift to competence-based training would be facilitated by the codification of observable behaviors, such as specific steps or errors, during an operation leading to assessment of performance.[11] Such behaviors during surgery relate not only to physical interactions between trainee, instruments, and the patient but also to communication, teamwork, and actions aimed at patient safety.[11]

In the future, a surgeon likely will see AI analysis of population and patient-specific data augmenting each phase of patient care. Automated analysis of all preoperative mobile and clinical data could provide a more patient-specific risk score for operative planning and yield valuable predictors for postoperative care and outcomes. Surgeons could then augment their decision-making intraoperatively based on real-time analysis of intraoperative progress that integrates electronic health data with operative video clips, vital signs, and instrument and hand tracking. Intraoperative monitoring of all available data could lead to timely prediction and avoidance of adverse events. Thus, with AI technologies, integration of preoperative, intraoperative, and postoperative data could lead to greater efficiency in predicting complications and improved patient recovery.

Although many feared that the threat of AI technologies is sentient self-awareness followed by an uprising of the machines as foretold by many futurists, this scenario is unlikely in the medical applications of AI, at least in the foreseeable future. Far more probable is that by the time AI and the appropriate user interfaces reach the proficiency level sufficient to replace human surgical educators, the practice of medicine will have evolved to the point where open surgery itself may be considered obsolete. Until such a time is realized, however, the role for AI -based education is rife with opportunity and holds potential for improving how surgeons develop and practice.

REFERENCES

1. Russell S, Bohannon J. Artificial intelligence. Fears of an AI pioneer. Science 2015;349(6245):252.
2. McKinsey Global Institute. Artificial intelligence: the next digital frontier? Discussion paper. 2017. Available at: https://www.mckinsey.com/~/media/mckinsey/industries/advanced%20electronics/our%20insights/how%20artificial%20intelligence%20can%20deliver%20real%20value%20to%20companies/mgi-artificial-intelligence-discussion-paper.ashx. Accessed February 15, 2019.
3. Johnson KW, Torres Soto J, Glicksberg BS, et al. Artificial intelligence in cardiology. J Am Coll Cardiol 2018;71:2668–79.
4. Kittanawong C, Zhang HJ, Wang Z, et al. Artificial intelligence in precision cardiovascular medicine. J Am Coll Cardiol 2017;69:2657–64.
5. Hashimoto DA, Rosman G, Rus D, et al. Artificial intelligence in surgery: promises and perils. Ann Surg 2018;268:70–6.
6. He J, Baxter SL, Xu J, et al. The practical implementation of artificial intelligence technologies in medicine. Nat Med 2019;25:30–6.

7. Dhindsa K, Bhandari M, Sonnadara RR. What's holding up the big data revolution in healthcare? Poor data quality, incompatible datasets, inadequate expertise, and hype. BMJ 2018;363:1–2.

8. Mirnezami R, Ahmed A. Surgery 3.0, artificial intelligence and the next-generation surgeon. Br J Surg 2018;105:463–5.

9. Bur AM, Shew M, New J. Artificial intelligence for the otolaryngologist: a state of the art review. Otolaryngol Head Neck Surg 2019;160(4):603–11.

10. Chan S, Siegel EL. Will machine learning end the viability of radiology as a thriving medical specialty? Br J Radiol 2019;92(1094):20180416.

11. Shorten G, Srinivasan K, Reinertsen I. Machine learning and evidence-based training in technical skills. Br J Anaesth 2018;121:521–3.

12. Deo RC. Machine learning in medicine. Circulation 2015;132:1920–30.

13. Esteva A, Robicquet A, Ramsunder B, et al. A guide to deep learning in healthcare. Nat Med 2019;25: 24–9.

14. Russell SJ, Norvig P. Artificial intelligence: a modern approach. 2nd edition. Upper Saddle River (NJ): Prentice Hall; 2003.

15. Poole DL, Mackworth AK. Artificial intelligence: foundations of computational agents. Cambridge (United Kingdom): Cambridge University Press; 2010.

16. Dartmouth Workship: Dartmouth Summer Research Project on Artificial Intelligence. Available at: https://en.wikipedia.org/wiki/Dartmouth_workshop. Accessed February 17, 2019.

17. Samuel AL. Some Studies in machine learning using the game of checkers. IBM Journal of Research and Development 1959;3:535–54.

18. Komura D, Ishikawa S. Machine learning methods for histopathological image analysis. Comput Struct Biotechnol J 2018;16:34–42.

19. Bejnordi EB, Veta M, Johannes van Diest P, et al. Diagnostic assessment of deep learning algorithms for detection of lymph node metastases in women with breast cancer. JAMA 2017;318:2199–210.

20. Wang X, Peng Y, Lu L, et al. ChestX-ray8: hospital-scale chest x-ray database and benchmarks on weakly supervised classification and localization of common thoracic diseases. Available at: https://arxiv.org/abs/1705.02315v4. Accessed February 20, 2019.

21. Gulshan V, Peng L, Coram M, et al. Development and validation of a deep learning algorithm for detection of diabetic retinopathy in retinal fundus photographs. JAMA 2016;316:2402–10.

22. Jirapatnakul AC, Fotin SV, Reeves AP, et al. Automated nodule location and size estimation using a multi-scale Laplacian of Gaussian filtering approach. Conf Proc IEEE Eng Med Biol Soc 2009; 2009:1028–31.

23. Esteva A, Kuprel B, Novoa RA, et al. Dermatologist-level classification of skin cancer with deep neural networks. Nature 2017;542:115–8.

24. Hilton L. The artificial brain as doctor—AI equals dermatologists in identifying lesions. Medpage Today 2018. Available at: https://www.medpagetoday.com/dermatology/generaldermatology/70513. Accessed February 18, 2019.

25. Crowson MG, Ranisau J, Eskander A, et al. A contemporary review of machine learning in otolaryngology–head and neck surgery. Laryngoscope 2019;00:1–7.

26. The AI effect. Available at: https://en.wikipedia.org/wiki/AI_effect. Accessed February 17, 2019.

27. Hu Z, Simon GJ, Arsoniadis EG, et al. Automated detection of postoperative surgical site infections using supervised methods with electronic health record data. Stud Health Technol Inform 2015;216: 706–10.

28. Soguero-Ruiz C, Fei WM, Jenssen R, et al. Data-driven temporal prediction of surgical site infection. AMIA Annu Symp Proc 2015;2015: 1164–73.

29. Bothe MK, Dickens L, Reichel K, et al. The use of reinforcement learning algorithms to meet the challenges of an artificial pancreas. Expert Rev Med Devices 2013;10:661–73.

30. Medved D, Ohlsson M, Höglund P, et al. Improving prediction of heart transplantation outcome using deep learning techniques. Sci Rep 2018;8:3613.

31. Soguero-Ruiz C, Hindberg K, Rojo-Alvarez JL, et al. Support vector feature selection for early detection of anastomosis leakage from bag-of-words in electronic health records. IEEE J Biomed Health Inform 2016;20:1404–15.

32. US Food and Drug Administration. FDA permits marketing of artificial intelligence-based device to detect certain diabetes related eye problems. Available at: https://www.fda.gov/newsevents/newsroom/pressannouncements/ucm604357.htm. Accessed February 20, 2019.

33. Richter R. Superstar Young scientist helps design software that measures a surgeon's skill. Stanford Medicine; 2018. Available at: http://stanmed.stanford.edu/2018fall/young-scientist-artificial-intelligence-measures-surgeons-skill.html. Accessed February 18, 2019.

34. Oakden-Rayner L. Exploring the ChestXray14 dataset: problems. Available at: https://lukeoakdenrayner.wordpress.com/2017/12/18/the-chestxray14-dataset-problems/. Accessed February 18, 2019.

35. Chan M, Esteve D, Fourniols JY, et al. Smart wearable systems: current status and future challenges. Artif Intell Med 2012;56:137–56.

36. Mitsuno D, Ueda K, Hirota Y, et al. Effective application of mixed reality device Hololens: Simple manual

alignment of surgical field and holograms. Plast Reconstr Surg 2019;143:647–51.

37. Brewer ZE, Fann HC, Ogden WD, et al. Inheriting the learner's view: a google glass-based wearable computing platform for improving surgical trainee performance. J Surg Educ 2016;73:682–8.

38. Mearian L. Did IBM overhype Watson Health's AI promise? Computerworld, November 14, 2018. Available at: https://www.computerworld.com/article/3321138/healthcare-it/did-ibm-put-too-much-stock-in-watson-health-too-soon.html. Accessed February 20, 2019.

Printed and bound by CPI Group (UK) Ltd, Croydon, CR0 4YY

08/05/2025

01864746-0013